TWO STEPS
FORWARD

Embracing life with a
brain tumor

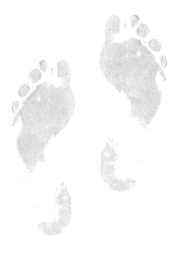

CLAIRE SNYMAN

Second printing, August 2022

ISBN 978-0-9947596-1-0
Ebook ISBN 978-0-9947596-0-3

Two Steps Publishing,
a Division of Synapse Consulting Inc
P.O. Box 93053
West Vancouver, BC
V7W 3G4
Canada

www.twosteps.ca

Edited by Pat Dobie.

Book cover design by Madeeha Shaikh, DezignManiac, Freelance Designer @ 99designs.com.

Book design and layout by Blush Book Design

Ebook edition by Bright Wing Books.

Legal Disclaimer

This book is not intended as a substitute for the medical advice of physicians. The eader should regularly consult a physician in matters relating to his/her health and particularly with respect to any symptoms that may require diagnosis or medical attention.

Internet references used in this work may have changed or disappeared between when this work was written and when it is read.

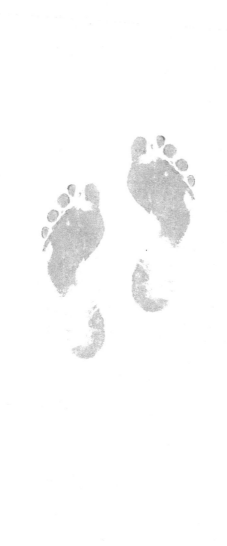

CONTENTS

This book is dedicated to my husband. Thank you for never giving up on me no matter what, and for standing by me. I am grateful each and every day for having you by my side. There is nowhere else I would rather be.

Acknowledgements

To my son Aiden, whose patience and sense of humor have helped me see the lighter side of things through this journey. I am forever grateful.

To my parents, who were there for us when we needed it most, as well as always being supportive and loving – I will never forget this.

To my family and friends who have helped in whatever way possible, I appreciate all you've done: the card sent, the phone call or email, the ear to listen, the dropped off dinner or the play date organized for Aiden.

To my General Practitioners, Dr. Seliske and Dr. Bujega, and to my neurosurgeon Dr. Alfredo Quiñones-Hinojosa, without whom I might not be where I am today. Dr. Q, you inspired me on so many levels and continue to do so today. Thank you as well to Dr. Toyota for his continued assistance in my care on many levels.

Also to the many survivors and patients with brain tumors, both non-malignant and malignant, you are my inspiration for sharing these words.

Additional thanks:

To the Colloid Cyst Survivors Facebook group: Your endless support and informative discussions made me feel I was not alone. Our shared experiences and questions prompted me to make this book a reality, in the hope that it may make just one person's journey a little easier.

To Sophia, my psychologist, who suggested that my thoughts and words could not only help me as an emotional outlet and healer, but might also help others.

To Pat, my editor, who took my words and helped them grow from being a fledgling to having the wings to fly and leave the nest. To Nicole, Melissa and Carita and my Mom for all their time taken in reviewing my manuscript and helping it along its way to being published. Thank you all.

PREFACE

MIRACLES

WHAT IS THE GREATEST MIRACLE? IT IS NOT WHAT I DO as a brain surgeon, but rather what my patients and families do when they put their lives or the lives of their loved ones in my hands. If I did not recognize that my patients and their families are performing miracles every day when they put their trust and hope in me, I would be failing to acknowledge one of life's truest, most amazing miracles.

Claire has done exactly that. Through her work and through her words she is giving so many patients the hope and strength to keep fighting despite the danger and despite the fact that sometimes, the odds may not be in their favor.

I remember the day that Claire and I went into the operating room to face this lesion right at the center of her brain—a cyst that was obstructing the flow of fluids in her brain and putting her life in danger. We did not know what to expect and we did not know what this lesion was, although we had an idea that it was a colloid cyst (a small "balloon" that was inflating into an area that would block the natural plumbing system of Claire's brain). But it easily could have been something completely different and more devastating, like a form of cancer. This possibility weighs heavily on patients and families, and is perhaps the most difficult part of my job, since I am often the one to carry the bad news. We went into the OR, but we did not go in alone. We had a team that was comprised of Claire's family and our anesthesiologists, nurses, technicians, neurologists, and many more health care providers amounting to no less than several dozen people orchestrating this surgery. Claire was at the top leading us, and I was her co-captain. Our team performs miracles like this every day by co-ordinating a complex orchestra that ensures the greatest outcome for our patients. They are in and out, and hopefully – like Claire – awake, alert, and doing well.

Claire is a natural leader and an inspirational role model. She guided us with her strength and allowed us to perform a miracle—to navigate the brain from the inside, just like one might imagine in a sci-fi movie, with small cameras and pieces of equipment that are smaller than the tips of pencils.

Claire's book is a testament to what the human spirit can do. She recollects her experiences with a passion and elegance, but at the same time with the strength that characterized her journey from diagnosis, to neurological compromise, to treatment, and towards recovery. You will not only relate to the anxieties of undergoing a surgery, and feel your own heart racing, but you will also come to understand the pain that Claire went through during her diagnosis and management, despite the fact that she remained strong and calm during the storm. Her recovery is remarkable, her words are deep, and her view of life is nothing short of heart warming—she is the real miracle!

It has been a privilege for me to be part of Claire's team. Claire may think that I was the leader of the team that brought her through the operation safely, but the truth is that she guided me during this journey, and she continues to guide me towards becoming a better physician, surgeon, and scientist—it is the greatest gift someone like me can receive.

Alfredo Quiñones-Hinojosa, *MD, FAANS, FACS*
William J. and Charles H. Mayo Professor
Chair, Neurologic Surgery
Mayo Clinic, Jacksonville, Florida, USA

Author's Note

This journey started in words as I realized that the time had come for me to put all my feelings— my happiness, blessings, gratitude, anger and fear—down somewhere where I would not be judged for what I was feeling and for the things that I said. The hardest part of my journey has been that while I physically look fine, my body and mind feel like they have been through a minefield. As time has passed, people, understandably, forget what has happened, even though it is sometimes as vivid as yesterday to me.

As time went by after my surgery and my strength returned, I remembered the turbulent time following my diagnosis: my uncertainty and fear, and my search for information. Therefore, I have decided to put my words and thoughts down, so that if there is just one person whom I can help and reassure with my words, then it is worth it.

Life with a brain tumor and life after brain surgery can be unexpected in so many ways. This book opens the door on the frustration, challenges and successes I faced both before and after my brain surgery and shows how this experience has changed my life and perspective forever.

And so...this is the story of a woman who lives most of her days realizing how blessed and grateful she is to be here in this moment, to have survived and be lucky enough to have only 'minor' setbacks from her surgery and condition. This woman also has some days, l ess often, where the frustrations of those minor setbacks seem overwhelming and she wonders when life will return to 'normal.' When will she stop taking steps backwards, and only start taking steps forwards? But the biggest lesson she has learned is that although there might be a step backward, she will always move forward, two steps forward. She must believe and remember this.

TO THE READER

To those who are reaching for this book as an **individual with a brain tumor**, I hope this helps you find one answer to a question you are looking for in your journey ahead. Strength to you, my friend.

To those who are reaching for this book as a **caregiver, spouse or loved one** of a person with a brain tumor, I hope this gives you insight into some of the thoughts, challenges and rewards along the way. You are the people those of us with brain tumors cannot do without. Thank you for your patience, love and care.

To those who are reaching for this book as a **medical professional**, I hope this helps you gain more of an understanding of the thoughts and feelings of a person with a brain tumor and those undergoing brain surgery, the 'behind-the-scenes' information that may not be found in a textbook. Thank you for your medical and emotional care of patients such as me. Please don't stop!

To those who are reaching for this book as a **general read**, I hope this book leaves you with a will to be your own advocate, make time your friend and to breathe in the small things in life.

One

SHOCKWAVE

May 14

Stop spinning, is my first thought. As my head comes off the pillow on waking, the light fixture above me is moving in circles. This is crazy...let me stand up. Not a good idea...this is worse than having drunk too much wine without enjoying the occasion. What is going on? Oh my goodness, I feel sick. Sick to my stomach. It is 6 am, according to my phone, which lies dancing on the bedside table beside me.

I cannot stand up without holding onto something, or the merry-go-round makes me fall over. I stumble to the washroom just in time and grasp the toilet bowl as the room continues to spin around me. It is early morning and I can hear the sounds of life downstairs. I feel terrible. I am normally a get-up-and-go person. Normally the alarm goes off and I am out of bed. Not this morning.

It is only twenty minutes later per the clock, but it feels like hours to me. The room is starting to spin at a slower rate, but the nausea still clings to me like a sheen of sweat. I stumble downstairs, hanging on to

1

the stair railing, to tell my husband, Marchand, that work is definitely a no go for me today. It must be some virus, and please can he take our four-year-old son to preschool? Okay, time to get to bed and sleep this off...except that lying down seems to make the spinning worse. I cling to the side of the bed like a life raft. The overhead light hanging from the ceiling becomes my point of focus, the compass that tells me that things are slowing down and the room is spinning slower. My exhausted body takes over, my eyes close and I sleep...

When I wake I am still feeling very lethargic, as if I have just completed a half marathon. Gee whiz, that was not a great introduction to vertigo—assuming that is what it was. I am hoping that is the last that I see of it! It must be a combination of this virus as well as just being really busy. I work full time as the international marketing manager at a local biotech company. I love my job. I love being a mom and a wife. But I am tired overall. This is probably just an accumulation of everything, my body's way of telling me to look at the stop sign in front of me. I am a perfectionist, a Type A personality, and always push myself to the limit, wanting to get everything and more done in the time frame I set myself. Not surprised that I feel so terrible today. It's been hectic!

May 17

After spending the last two days in bed recovering from that vertigo attack I have decided to visit my GP, as I have now developed a massive headache. The vertigo has gone, thank goodness, but I am still feeling off balance. I feel hungover. I have been working from home rather than heading into the office and infecting anyone else with whatever it is I am harboring in my body.

I have never been someone who suffers from headaches, so this is a new thing. My husband gets bad sinus headaches and migraines and I have never really understood how painful and debilitating they are. The "crawl into a dark room under the bed covers" advice seems absolutely right. The light is too bright for me; even the weak sunlight today is painful. My GP has advised that, given the sudden onset of all these symptoms and the fact that I have never been a headache sufferer, I should go to the local ER if it does not resolve over the next day.

May 18

I feel worse. My husband urges me to head straight to the ER. I call my doctor's office and they agree—they want me to be checked out for meningitis. So off I go. On arrival I explain that my GP thinks I might have meningitis. I am promptly handed a facemask. Funny how people don't sit next to you when you are wearing one of those blue masks. I don't care; I just want to feel better. I am admitted in the ER and my veins are exposed to needles for blood tests, as well as an IV to get some fluids coursing through my body. The doctor orders a CT (computerized tomography[1]) scan and a lumbar puncture to see if there is anything to explain the onset of these symptoms. As I am lying on the CT scan table, staring up at the roof, which has maple leaves on it, I think, what if I have something in my head that is not supposed to be there?

I am back in my ER bed, waiting for any news from the doctor, when my husband arrives. What a star he is. I wasn't expecting to see him. But I do feel relieved to have someone I know nearby. He heads off to get a quick coffee. I listen to what is going on around me in the ER: always so much on the go, patients talking, groaning, doctors, nurses, questions, answers. I hear the doctors talking down the hall about a brain tumor and saying that it is quite unusual and rare. There seem to be quite a few people discussing it and looking at the scans, and I think: "What a thing for that person". Little did I know that they were talking about me.

1   CT scan combines a series of X-ray views taken from many different angles and computer processing to create cross-sectional images of the bones and soft tissues inside your body http://www.mayoclinic.org/tests-procedures/ct-scan/basics/definition/p c-20014610

Tick tock, goes the slow clock inside the ER.

Eventually the doctor arrives to talk to me but Marchand is still out, so I am alone when the doctor tells me: "We still need to do a lumbar puncture to check for meningitis, but the CT scan found that you have a colloid cyst in your brain."

What? My heart stops. Are you kidding? A *what* in my brain?

"Don't worry," he says. "The colloid cyst is often an incidental finding and we don't think it is causing your symptoms, but we will get a neurosurgeon to come down and see you to chat further about managing it." And he leaves.

I take a deep breath. Oh my gosh. My pulse races. I pull out my phone—screw any rules about cell phones in the ER—and rapidly Google: Colloid Cyst. I scan the information and read that it is a non-malignant brain tumor of sorts in the third ventricle of the brain, and it can require brain surgery if it is problematic.

"Approximately three people per million per year receive a diagnosis of a colloid cyst,"[2] I read. "Approximately 0.1-1% of all primary brain tumors and 15-20% of all intraventricular masses are colloid cysts."[3] "On rare occasions, a colloid cyst may obstruct the foramen of Monro completely and irreversibly, resulting in sudden loss of consciousness and, if patients are not treated, coma and subsequent death due to herniation."[4]

That is all I can read before Marchand walks back in smiling with his coffee: "Any news?"

How do I do this? How do I tell my husband that I have a brain tumor, albeit non-malignant? I almost want to laugh. I am still digesting the information myself. So I just do it: "They think I may have viral meningitis and are going to do a lumbar puncture to check.

2   http://radiology.rsna.org/content/239/3/650.full
3   http://emedicine.medscape.com/article/249401-overview#a0199
4   http://emedicine.medscape.com/article/249401-overview#a0112

And they also found a brain tumor on the CT scan. It's not malignant." I stop. I just don't know what to do.

I see his eyes brim with tears. "You are kidding, right?"

I feel numb. Given that we know so little, there is no point in having a panic attack right now, so we wait. We just hold hands in silence and wait for the neurosurgeon. I lie there in the emergency room with a thousand thoughts flying through my mind. I oscillate between wanting to laugh hysterically or cry out loud.

Shortly thereafter, the doctor comes in to do my lumbar puncture and then we wait. About an hour later, we finally meet the neurosurgeon. A neurosurgeon has always been one of those godly specialists that I never thought I would have to meet, especially to have a look at my own brain. This seems surreal on so many levels. He tells us that I will have an MRI (magnetic resonance imaging[5]) in about two weeks, so they can see the cyst in more detail. He tell us that most people live their lives without ever having any issues with the cyst, and that they doubt my current symptoms are caused by it, although at one centimeter, it is medium to large in size.

They will monitor me yearly with MRIs to see if the cyst grows.

The lumbar puncture reveals that I most likely have viral meningitis. Viral meningitis has similar symptoms to bacterial meningitis but for the most part is not as deadly or as debilitating[6]. There is no specific treatment and I will just require rest and some tender loving care at home, then I should start to feel better.

Okay, let's go home. I feel numb, in my back from being stabbed for the lumbar puncture, in my arms from the drips, and in the rest of my body and mind from the shock of my other diagnosis.

---

5   MRI is a technique that uses a magnetic field and adio waves to create detailed images of the organs and tissues within your body. http://www.mayoclinic.org/tests-procedures/mri/basics/definition/p c-20012903

6   http://www.nmaus.org/disease-prevention-information/is-it-viral-bacterial-or-fungal/

I have been in the ER all day, so our kind neighbor has looked after Aiden and now our babysitter has tucked him up in bed. I walk in on him fast asleep and my heart feels torn in pieces as I see his little chest move up and down. My little man, only four years old, my miracle for whom I would do anything, lies blissfully unaware of the torment in my mind and heart.

I wait till the timing is decent and call my parents in South Africa, tens of thousands of kilometers away, to tell them about our day. I really don't have too much to tell them, given that I am still coming to terms with it and don't know more than what I was told today in the ER.

That night I search more online to understand what a colloid cyst is and what it means. There is not a load of information, but I hope the next weeks will reveal more information and medical research about this condition. It is now 11 pm and dark outside. I hold onto my husband like a life raft and let the flood of tears from the day pour down my face.

Two

CHANGE IS THE ONLY CONSTANT

MY NAME IS CLAIRE HELEN SNYMAN AND I AM THIRty-four years old. I feel, however, that I have lived a lifetime in the past eight years. I am South African by birth, have lived in Sydney, Australia for four years and now live in Vancouver, Canada—blessed with mountains, ocean, fresh air and Canadians. My husband and I moved here in 2006, when I was five months pregnant. What an adventure! Within four weeks of moving our worldly goods from a large container into our new home, our precious son Aiden decided to arrive four weeks early. I am sure he had had enough of my lifting, bending and moving-in antics and wanted out.

Well, motherhood was an introduction to my life's biggest adventure and still is. My personality that thrives on structure, routine and things going my way with hard work, was turned upside down and inside out. No books that I read—and believe me, I had read them all—could have taught me how to soothe a premature infant with bad reflux and a cow's milk protein allergy in the wee hours of the morning.

It is interesting that when you are pregnant, you read all these books about what to expect as a new parent, anything from breastfeeding to sleep training to toddler tantrums. By the time Aiden was born, I had read over ten books and felt ready to take on the role of parenthood. Unfortunately, I did not realize that there really is no book on parenthood; only the one that you write yourself as you go through the ever-changing days and years ahead.

I have now discovered that the one area that is not covered in the books is the change that can take place in your career and work life after having kids. Note: this is definitely a person-specific and situation-specific issue. I returned to work after eleven months of maternity leave and realized how much I had missed my work. This did make me feel guilty, now that I was a mom. I had always been a very career-focused individual. But after being at home with my son on maternity leave, I also really appreciated the chance to finish my cup of tea in the office in one sitting and not try and remember where in the house I had left it when being distracted from the opportunity to sip my life-renewing brew. I would also learn over the coming years that my career and life would morph, as my son grew older and changed from a toddler to a young boy and both of our needs changed.

For our family, change seems to be the one constant in our lives. If you had asked me when I met my husband where we would be living and bringing up our family, the obvious answer to me would have been South Africa. We are both South African and both our families are there. Yet here we are, living on the west coast of Canada. We are pretty much as far as we could be from our families, who live in Durban and Johannesburg, South Africa—them on the east coast of Africa and us on the west coast of Canada.

Times changed after we married, and we decided to move to Australia. We left both our families in South Africa and with four suitcases each and a house in a large container, we boarded the plane. We had no jobs waiting, only a booked accommodation for the first two weeks. And so the beginning of our life of change started.

Australia is an amazing country. I still remember the warmth, the kookaburras and lorikeets in the trees, the smell of eucalyptus in the heat and the blueness of the sky during the drought. We were extremely happy in Sydney; we had a good life there and very fond memories.

While there, we tried to get pregnant 'naturally.' I suffer from endometriosis and underwent two laparoscopies, then eventually we decided to try *in vitro* fertilization (IVF). I had a very low egg survival rate from the twelve harvested, so we were blessed that the one little egg that was implanted resulted in a pregnancy. Only two were 'viable'—the new life in my tummy and the other that we had cryo-preserved for the future. I will never forget that I was able to see our 'in-transit' embryo under the microscope before they implanted the egg. Only eight cells big as a blastocyst, and now that blastocyst had found a home.

Soon after the IVF, work called and Vancouver offered a new opportunity for my husband and for us as a new 'work-in-progress' family. I loved my job but was very newly pregnant and this seemed a good time to move, as I would soon be taking time off for maternity leave as well.

I had never even been to Canada before our first 'look-see' visit about nine months before we moved from Australia. Canada had always seemed like a foreign land to me, locked in ice drifts and snow. Ha! I was wrong, especially about Vancouver, which in the winter is the equivalent of the 'Bahamas' of Canada.

My background is in the medical and clinical field. I studied as a clinical dietitian in South Africa and spent my first job working in pediatrics at the largest hospital in the world, Chris Hani Baragwanath in Soweto.

For people who have never been to South Africa, Soweto stands for 'South Western Townships' and is home to about 1.3 million people.

Soweto consists of some areas of houses but the majority is made of "shanty houses" of corrugated iron strips somehow strapped together to form a shelter. Here, kids play in the dirt streets with an old soccer ball, often wearing torn shirts and clothes. Life is completely different from anything most of us have ever known.

Even for me, being South African, my eyes were opened wide during this work experience. My dad always said that I should go for this opportunity as it would 'grow hair on my teeth' and he was right! "Bara," as we called the hospital, was a great place to learn things not seen in the usual day-to-day medical profession. It was a great personal learning experience for me as well, to see that there was hope in such a desolate place.

The pediatric wards were my favorite place to be. A lot of the children were not visited on a daily basis by their parents, as the cost of getting transport to the hospital from their homes was too much on their meager salaries. Hence, I did all my responsibilities as a clinical dietitian ensuring that the kids who were being fed special diets or via NGT (nasogastric tube) or even parenterally (IV) were getting everything they needed. But I was also lucky enough to be able to spend a few extra minutes with special children, whom I still remember to this day. I'd give them a walk outside, a push on the old swing, or just a hug when they were crying. I wanted to take them all home with me at the end of the day.

I was also able to go into surgery with many of my patients and loved this. Even to this day, when Aiden and I play a card game that asks: "If you could do any job in the world for one day, what would you choose and why?" my answer is always, "A surgeon, because I love being in surgery (note, not as a patient and knowing that what you are doing can make an immediate difference in that person's life."

However, after being involved indirectly in a shoot-out at the hospital, I knew the time had come for me to try something different. My heart was still in the medical field; something about hospitals and the clinical field intrigued me. I continued my career into the pharmaceutical arena with a marketing degree and loved the combination of medical knowledge and business skills. My newfound passion was business development and product management. However, I firmly believe that there are certain jobs in one's life that are meant to teach you something. My job at Bara taught me empathy for people who had less than I did. To be exposed to the extreme end of poverty and harsh life that many families lived was a rude awakening. Even living in South Africa, a third world country, I did not see this end of the realm in my daily life, apart from beggars at the traffic lights or driving past the townships on my way to work.

Another job that was a learning experience for me was working at a pharmaceutical company in Australia and specializing in schizophrenia and bipolar disorders. My learning from this was profound. In my role as a clinical consultant, I visited acute mental health wards, prisons and more. I had not realized the prevalence of mental illness and the profound impact it can have on a person and their family; how people's lives can literally change overnight. What you see on the outside of a person is not necessarily what is going on inside. And at the same time, don't judge that person on the corner who is talking to the trees, dancing in the street or behaving strangely. Life might be dramatically different for them, far different from anything you know or understand.

One day I would remember these wise lessons.

Three

THE AFTERMATH

May 31

It is now two weeks post diagnosis.

Now that I have read up as much as I think I possibly can online regarding my colloid cyst, the biggest challenge for me is the mental and emotional part of the diagnosis, the part you don't find online or hear from your neurosurgeon. I am the mom of a four-year-old boy and my mind races with thoughts from the normal to the bizarre. The far end of it all is: What if I die? This is a rare brain tumor; do they really know everything there is to know about it? What if I start convulsing or having other severe symptoms? How will this impact my family, my husband, my son and me?

Looking back, I remembered seeing my GP two years earlier, as I felt like my short-term memory was being affected. I was not able to remember things like I used to. We did a few memory tests and put it down to being a full-time working mom who had a two-year-old child. Was this a sign?

I cannot seem to work through if how I am feeling is related to my body reacting to the news of my diagnosis, or to the viral meningitis, or to the cyst—it is just all so confusing. I cannot seem to compartmentalize things yet.

From my extensive online search it seems like the most common symptoms of a colloid cyst are:

> Headache, gait disturbances, short-term memory loss, nausea, vomiting, behavioral changes. Sudden weakness in the lower limbs associated with falls and without loss of consciousness (drop attacks) have been reported. An alternative theory suggests that sudden death in patients with colloid cysts may be related to acute neurogenic cardiac dysfunction (secondary to the acute hydrocephalus) and subsequent cardiac arrest rather than herniation.[7]

A couple of years later, I would be part of a survey of over two hundred of our Colloid Cyst Survivors Facebook group and we would see that most of us prior to surgery suffered from a mix of headaches/migraines, dizziness/vertigo, a feeling of imbalance, visual disturbances, fatigue, short-term memory loss, depression and anxiety/panic attacks and tinnitus (ringing in ears) as the most common symptoms experienced. This symptom profile tended to follow that of non-malignant brain tumors in general.

One of the best definitions I would hear, almost one and a half years after surgery, was that "a colloid cyst is a non-malignant tumor in a malignant location." Absolutely spot on.

Right, so the general symptoms of headache and nausea seem okay but the others of short-term memory loss, behavioral changes and sudden death, freak me out completely.

---

7 http://emedicine.medscape.com/article/249401-overview#a0112. Note: this information is from an online search and is intended to be a quick brush stroke overview. Consult your neurosurgeon or neurologist for further information.

So, my colloid cyst is a rare, congenital (present from birth slow growing neoplasm or tumor. It is made up of a gel like material and it seems like the onset of symptoms for most people is usually between twenty to fifty years of age although some people go through life never even knowing they ever had one [8].

The great thing about the Internet is the accessibility to data and information. The not-so-great thing about the Internet is the accessibility to data and information. Too much information makes my head spin. It feels like I have a little time bomb inside my head with a detonator programmed to go off, but no one knows when.

Looking back many months after my diagnosis had set in, I realized that this was actually the hardest part of the whole situation: the not knowing if symptoms were related to my colloid cyst or not. Learning how to deal with this reality—to live with it, feel comfortable with it, and not let it take over my life or become an obsession—was a hard lesson.

Having a cyst in your brain might not be considered a 'big deal' by some health care professionals, and they can be dismissive. The other challenge is that having a non-malignant brain tumor does not always require immediate treatment, but rather a 'watch and wait' approach. Looking back, I think the best way for me personally to deal with it was to feel confident in the medical opinion around me and the consensus of my treating doctors. If they were confident and happy, I felt confident and happy. I also learned which symptoms meant I needed to seek further attention i.e. a headache that would not go away after my normal migraine medication regime. However, later in my journey, the medical opinion around me did not sync with my own personal opinion and the opinion that I had researched. I sought a second opinion, which might have saved my life. So a note to self that I still firmly believe in to this day: Be your own advocate and learn to listen to your own body.

---

8 Turillazzi, Emanuela et al. "Colloid Cyst of the Third Ventricle, Hypothalamus, and Heart: a Dangerous Link for Sudden Death." Diagnostic Pathology 7 (2012): 144. PMC. Web. 16 Feb. 2015.

I have told only my immediate bosses at work about my brain situation. I have been off work now for about two weeks, recovering from the viral meningitis. Marchand has been an incredible support, helping me out as he knows I am still so tired, but also as he knows I am not quite sure how to deal with this all. Trying to make heads and tales of this situation is like playing Pickup Sticks. I am not quite sure how he is able to deal with this. He has always been remarkably strong when it comes to situations that are crisis-driven and that require acute focus. I could not love him more than I do at this moment.

It feels like a lifetime has happened over the past two weeks of being at home. Now it is time to head back to work and act as if everything is normal and I was just recovering from viral meningitis.

I don't want people to know what is going on. Work is extremely important to me and I want my role within the office to continue to be based on my competencies and have nothing to do with my condition. It is better this way.

June 2

My second day back in the office. But it is hard for me to get back into the swing of things. Some things just seem mundane. There are moments when I must leave the office before my tears of confusion overwhelm me. I take a walk to the local coffee shop, grab a tea and then call my mom, thousands of miles away. It's probably a thoroughly indecent time there, but I need to hear her voice. I want her to reassure me that it's going to be okay. I have not broadcasted the news of the past weeks to many people, just my close friends who knew I had been ill and not my normal self.

Even for a thirty-four-year-old woman there is something very comforting about hearing your mother's voice telling you that it is okay to cry and to feel uncertain, and that she is there to listen. Once the tears stop, I take a deep breath and walk back to the office of normalcy.

The Aftermath

I have been told that my colloid cyst is most likely an incidental find
ing. Incidental is defined as occurring merely by chance, or without
intention or calculation. So this means that the chances that the new
onset of headaches or migraines and vertigo is highly unlikely to be
related to my colloid cyst.

To be honest, although I have no medical degree, I feel that this does
not make sense. I have never suffered from headaches of any nature
my whole life and now, at the age of thirty-four, have started suffering
from migraines and vertigo and, lo and behold, they found a one-
centimeter colloid cyst in my brain. How can these not be related?

Since my vertigo attack I have also been suffering from what I
have called 'out-of-body' experiences. I feel like my energy and
spirit is literally being drained from my body. A numbness starts in
my face and seeps through my body, as if all my blood is being
drained onto the floor. I feel as if I am walking on clouds, observing
my body from a distance. I also cannot tolerate bright light, and I
still get the odd feeling of vertigo.

I have started to keep a diary of when I get migraines, vertigo or any
of these weird experiences as my memory seems like a fog. I think
this is a good idea for anyone diagnosed with a new condition that
seems to be a bit overwhelming in the beginning. Keeping a diary of
how you are feeling helps when you go to see the doctor. It also
allows you to put down questions in one place so you will
remember to ask the doctor. Somehow, being in front of a doctor
can put you on the spot and you forget all the questions you meant
to ask, then you walk out kicking yourself. I think I am now a doctor's
worst nightmare as I walk in with a list of typed questions. But hey,
that is how I ensure that I know all my avenues are covered.

I have now received my date for my first MRI in order for them to see
the cyst in more detail. I have also been referred to a neurologist as I
am still suffering from bad headaches, three weeks after the first one

occurred. The neurologist said that the meningitis might continue to give me headaches for quite a while. He had seen a few young women recently with this situation take up to six months to feel back to normal. So I leave with a script for a migraine medication, Axert[9] and a follow up appointment. He also notes that I do have an element of vestibular dysfunction, which could account for the vertigo attack I experienced.

June 6

I am back in the ER again as my migraines are still not resolving. It is now almost four weeks since my diagnosis. They find nothing indicative of any changes in the ER and since I have an MRI scheduled this week and my neurosurgical consult, it seems everything is lined up to ensure I am being cared for.

I had yet to realize that this would become a key part of dealing with my colloid cyst in the future; knowing how to deal with the emotions and sense of dread and uncertainty that would come with having a headache and migraine. Is it the cyst, is my brain swelling or is it just a headache, a normal headache. What is a normal headache, or a migraine? Every time I mentioned it to my neurosurgeon or neurologist, I was told the headaches had nothing to do with my cyst. "Her current presentation is unlikely related to ventricular obstruction in association with her colloid cyst". I think it is a hard thing to tell a patient who has a brain tumor that it may or may not result in a condition such as hydrocephalus (buildup of fluid in the cavities (ventricles) deep within the brain[10]), which may be like a massive headache, and not expect them to feel anxious about normal headaches coming and going.

---

9   Note: any medication referred to here is based off my individual medical history and medical visit.
10   http://www.mayoclinic.org/diseases-conditions/hydrocephalus/basics/definition/con-2003070

June 9

My first MRI was today. I had no idea what to expect. I have only ever had a CT scan done before when they found the colloid cyst. Today they did the MRI with and without contrast, which meant I had an IV line placed, which I did not realize would be done. Probably better that way. The MRI machine is a lot louder that I ever expected and they give you earplugs for it because of all the loud clonking and going on. It took about an hour in total with short spurts of lying absolutely still for the images to be taken. Although I thought I would feel claustrophobic when I saw the machine, I actually felt okay. My head felt sore being held in place in a metal box with cushioning to ensure I did not move an inch. Well, it is now done and we will get the results at my neurosurgeon's appointment this week.

June 11

Today we have my first appointment with my neurosurgeon. He shares the results from my first MRI which show the colloid cyst at 1.2 centimeters and no sign of hydrocephalus or ventricular enlargement. My neurosurgeon explains to Marchand and I that it is a moderately large cyst, hence we can, if we want, consider the option of surgical removal given the potential for it to grow and cause problems with ventricular obstruction.

He does not know if the removal of the cyst will result in any improvement of my headache symptoms, though. He also explains the risks, benefits and expectations associated with surgical intervention. We decide to reassess and monitor the cyst with annual MRIs for the time being. I will continue to see the neurologist for monitoring and treatment of my migraines and see the neurosurgeon again in one year for another MRI and follow up.

The thought of brain surgery sends shivers down my spine. I have been through many other surgeries in the past, but something about brain surgery just seems too extreme for me at this point in time. We join the 'watch and wait' group of brain tumor patients around the world.

July 22

Now that more time has passed since my diagnosis and now that I am in the health care system and being monitored, I am starting to feel more at ease and not as overwhelmed. I have also found a Facebook group for colloid cyst survivors, which I join. I am still reading up as much as I can to understand this rare condition. It can, however, be very overwhelming, even depressing, reading people's encounters with a colloid cyst, having brain surgery and especially post-operative symptoms and outcomes. Not that I don't want to know about post-surgery issues, I just need to breathe for a while. I think I may have overloaded myself with information.

August 3

I am scheduled for a second MRI, as my headaches and vertigo are not resolving. So off I go again.

The neurologist calls me to tell me the results. He says that everything looks fine with the cyst and that there's no ventricular enlargement, however they have noticed a new white spot on the MRI. I apparently had a few of them before, but have a new one now. He has consulted with a Multiple Sclerosis (MS) specialist and they both agreed that this white spot is in no way related to MS. My heart does a double flip. I know what MS is all about. But they seem to have done their homework and ruled that out.

The past months have been stressful for us as a family and we are ready for some rest and relaxation. We head off to California for some well overdue leave and sun! Since a colloid cyst seems to be such a rare condition, that three-in-a-million chance, we consider seeing a neurosurgeon in Los Angeles while we're there.

We head off to the beaches, basking in the sun and enjoying being away. The huge and never-ending landscape of LA is overwhelming after living in Vancouver for so long. Back home, a highway that has over six lanes packed with cars in both directions is unheard of.

I do my online research to see what is available in LA and find the University of California, Los Angeles (UCLA), which has a good reputation. We are able to book an appointment to see a neurosurgeon there who has experience dealing with and removing colloid cysts. I see him and have another neurological evaluation—I'm getting so used to these I could do them in my sleep. Yes, my accounting skills are questionable when asked math questions and basic subtraction and addition, but I'm not sure I can blame that on the cyst!

His opinion takes us by surprise. Totally.

"If you were my wife, I would get this removed —this is going to cause you problems some day, maybe not tomorrow, but some day for sure. You are already showing subtle signs of the cyst impacting your brain. Given the size of your cyst, the natural history is that you will become symptomatic and it is best to remove this prior to any obstructive hydrocephalus occurring."

We leave shell-shocked. This is completely opposite to the opinions back home of "watch and wait." On the plane home we hold hands, not quite sure what to make of all the new information.

Once we are back in Vancouver and settled after our holiday away, I start to feel a need to get a local second opinion. I live in Canada, so I should really focus more on what the local opinion is, as this is where I would get surgery, right? It seems such a huge step to go and get brain surgery when I do not yet have any serious complications. My migraines and occasional 'out-of-body' experiences are the only symptoms I am having. And I've been told that these are not related to the cyst.

I feel like a hypochondriac, asking to get a second local opinion after just being in Los Angeles but we just don't feel 100 percent comfortable with the brain surgery opinion. So my GP arranges for me to see another neurosurgeon at the largest hospital in Vancouver. He is really professional and has a good reputation. He states that the current risks of brain surgery outweigh my risks from the colloid cyst at this point and that my ventricles are of a normal size. The serial MRIs are, however, very important for tracking the size and impact of the cyst on the brain, so I should continue with these at my local hospital.

Truth be told, I am not sure what prompts me to search for yet another opinion. The neurosurgeon in the United States said I should have it out immediately. Of the two local neurosurgeons, one stated that serial MRIs were mandatory, but both said that surgery was not necessary. I feel confused and, as a mother, maybe over-concerned. But, after chatting to my very objective husband, we agree that I would find out where the best neurosurgical hospital is in the United States and see what options they offer for external consults.

Given that the yearly incidence of a colloid cyst is three people per million, my one thought is that maybe I need to look to a hospital that has a large patient population both locally and internationally. This is my brain, after all, that we are talking about. So, after lots of searching and reading online, I am able to secure an external consult at Johns Hopkins Hospital, Baltimore.

US News & World Report has consistently ranked Johns Hopkins as the number one institution in the United States for neurosurgery and neurology. They also have a very large international base of patients, so this would be a good place to get a consult, as they should have a good number of colloid cysts floating through their doors. Having worked in the pharmaceutical and medical device industry and being a health care professional myself, I know that this hospital has a stellar reputation.

I send through all my MRIs and complete all the required information forms. The procedure is that they review all your medical forms and MRIs, and then they call you to discuss your case. They are very professional and the final verdict is absolutely to have serial MRIs, just as you would have your blood pressure tested if you have a blood pressure issue.

This is how I met the neurosurgeon who would eventually make a huge impact, in more ways than one, on my life: Dr. Alfredo Quinones-Hinojosa (also known as Dr. Q.) Dr. Q states that the colloid cyst is not a surgical issue at present but that I must ensure I am doing the yearly MRIs to ensure this does not change.

I now feel like I have covered all my bases. I feel reassured and happy with the care I am receiving locally. Yes, it may seem over dramatic, but I have had conflicting reviews from two doctors and just wanted to be sure.

When you have a condition that is rare, you need to be your own advocate and pursue all avenues, if you can, to get the answers you need to feel comfortable with the care you have. Even specialists do not see rare conditions every day, every year. They may only see a couple a year, if that many. Continue to be your own advocate.

Four

LIFE IN BETWEEN

June 14

It is now over a year since I was diagnosed. Time has flown. I still continue to suffer from migraines; I also have a feeling of 'blurring' in one eye. I feel like bits of my vision are missing and I sometimes do need to focus more clearly. I have seen an ophthalmologist but have been given the all clear. Otherwise: healthy and happy.

Since being diagnosed I have found that my priorities have changed. I still work as hard as I used to, but it has dawned on me that I would like to spend more time at home with Aiden. I am lucky enough to be able to take a step back and go from working five days a week to working three days a week. This means I can spend Fridays and Mondays at home with my son.

The past year has highlighted to me the importance of being in the moment and making the most of things, the most of life. I need to be in the moment with my son and watch him grow; he is at that stage that is great to be a part of. My four-year-old son is growing up so fast and I feel I may blink and miss it. I am still super busy at work, loving my job but also enjoying being at home with Aiden the extra two days a week now even though I still seem to do some work on my days off too. But that could also just be me, trying to get everything done all at once.

This year has been one to remember, a place marker in my life. I now feel more in control of everything. I no longer get that sense of dread when I get a migraine. I just take my medication and wait it out. I know I have a non-malignant tumor in my brain but I have decided it is not going to get in the way of my life. However, it has been a lesson learned for sure, and it has not been an easy one or an overnight one. I certainly look at things differently now. I hold moments dearer than I used to. This has been a good lesson for me, I think for us all.

I know I am blessed with my husband, my son, family, great friends, and a job I love. We live in a great country, too. Some people still ask me if we are ever going to have another child. I just tell them that I think my body has told me that it could not head down that road again, too much has happened and we have one miracle already, for which we are blessed.

It is true about reassessing one's life when you get a curveball thrown at you. The past ten years or so have been a struggle for my body health wise. My body just seems to have lots of things happen to it even though I consider myself to be genuinely healthy as a person. As we joke, my warranty does not seem to have enough years on it! But I am determined to not let this new situation win!

The truth about the change in life hits me again. I am clocking in over ten hours a day, four days a week, even though I am supposed to be working three. This may not seem excessive work to some people but I am questioning myself. Is this really what I want right now?

Eventually, I think about this with my heart. Aiden is heading off to kindergarten this September and I would like to be part of that transition, but I'm not sure how that would work if I were still working the 'normal' office based job. I also question how we are going to manage the intense ten-week summer holidays when I get only two to three weeks leave a year.

I think long and hard about this, and decide the time has come to try and do something on my own. So, with a sad and uncertain feeling, I quit my job to start my own consulting business in marketing and business development. Once again, change seems to be the only constant in our lives!

July 15

It is that time of year again when I head off into the loud metal tube for my annual MRI. As I insert earplugs in my ears, that sense of uncertainty hits me. A shiver of fear runs through me as I wonder what they will find this time around. It always feels like a game of Russian roulette.

At my visit to the neurologist I get the follow-up news on my MRI. Well, they confirm I have a brain, which is excellent news. There is nothing noticeable regarding any impact from the colloid cyst on the surrounding areas of the brain. My colloid cyst is still approximately 1.2 centimeters and stable, with no sign of obstructive hydrocephalus. I feel like I have passed a test with flying colors! My neurologist says that it is no longer necessary to follow me with serial MRIs. However, if I were to have any new or progressive symptoms, they would revisit the issue.

I automatically assume this is a decision he and my neurosurgeon have decided upon together, as he has copied my neurosurgeon on his report. My first feeling is of great relief and excitement. I call my husband to tell him. This is good news. Until it settled in and I thought about it a bit more. This was contrary to the two opinions I had recently received where serial MRIs were considered proper and mandatory treatment to monitor the status of the colloid cyst.

One neurosurgeon explained it to me as saying "if you had diabetes, you would monitor your blood glucose, if you had high blood pressure, you would monitor your blood pressure. There is no way of saying that the cyst is stable or that symptoms are not related unless you do annual MRIs so we have something to compare to." This same neurosurgeon said that if I went for a couple of years with no change or growth, then I might be able to go for an MRI every two years. He didn't suggest abrupt cessation of imaging.

I feel uncomfortable. What now? This has undermined my faith in these two health care professionals. Well, I have the consult and relationship with the neurosurgeon at Johns Hopkins and am very happy with him, so I could keep that going and be monitored with him and his team. It is a fine balance between feeling like a hypochondriac and feeling like you need more information or don't feel 100 percent confident in your current medical opinion.

Just to be sure, I send my contact neurosurgeon at Johns Hopkins an email and ask his opinion about stopping my MRIs. He replies that I absolutely need to continue the yearly MRIs and adds that he would be happy to carry on monitoring me.

Given that this is my brain, we feel comfortable continuing care at Johns Hopkins. It is easy enough to be followed up remotely at Johns Hopkins as a patient. So we make the decision. At this stage it only involves getting my MRIs done here locally and sending them to the United States for review, nothing that cannot be handled by the postal system. We are sorted out!

This would be my first in many lessons of learning to be my body's own advocate.

One of the other things to get ticked off my medical list at the moment is my ears. In Australia, about three months into my pregnancy I developed a ringing noise known as tinnitus in both of my ears. As I was pregnant they could not do an MRI as part of the normal medical work up in Australia. Since arriving in Canada, having a baby, going back to work and settling in, and life just passing us by, I have mostly ignored it. The ringing is always there, but increases if I am stressed. Now, almost six years later, I feel like my hearing is not as good as it should be, especially in crowded rooms or a restaurant. I sometimes struggle to hear everything people are saying.

A hearing test and visit to the ENT (ear, nose and throat surgeon) show I have a mild hearing loss in my left ear and the tinnitus also does not help my hearing at the high-level frequency. My ENT suggests that I ensure people are in front of me when talking, not in the next room, so that lip reading and visibility can help me make sense of the words. This suggestion seems valid and is a good reason as to why my son cannot talk to me from upstairs and assume I hear what he is saying (as most kids assume at this age). Oh well, can tick the done box now – tick!

Later, a significant percentage of colloid cyst patients in our Facebook group survey would show they too had tinnitus prior to surgery. Interesting, hmmm?

December 9

The time of year has come for us to make like swallows and migrate to the southern hemisphere. I am so excited. We are going back to South Africa for a well-overdue holiday. Great timing, as this tends to be a tricky time of year in Vancouver. The rain is here, the snow for ski season is not quite on the local mountains, so a sunny vacation will be most welcome.

The best part is being able to spend quality time with our families. Being so far away becomes acutely obvious during these times, so we lap it all up during these holidays. Bliss!

On arrival in South Africa we feel like we have circumnavigated the globe. Two long-haul flights and about thirty-five hours door to door, but we eventually arrive in Cape Town to glorious blue skies and baking hot weather. After very little sleep, my son finds his swim gear, snorkel and flippers, stands ready and announces he is ready to swim. This brings a smile to my weary face. We go outside into the vitamin D-enriched rays and soak up the sun, the energy and warmth. Bliss, after the rain-soaked clouds of Vancouver.

We spend four wonderful weeks in South Africa in Cape Town and in KwaZulu-Natal with our families, swimming, walking, talking and just enjoying the lazy summer days. Christmas brings back so many memories of my childhood. A southern hemisphere Christmas, spent outside, swimming in a pool or at the beach with an ice cream in hand. Aiden's main concern was whether Santa would know where to find him.

Every morning Marchand and I would go walking or running before the swelter of the morning heat descended and it was too hot to do any exercise. It's a wonderful feeling to be out there in the early hours of the day and feel the heat on your shoulders, the sweat begin to drip down your body. There is something amazingly special about the beaches in South Africa, the raw intensity of the crashing waves, the white rush of the waves over the sand.

Some evenings we would go down to the beach as a family and sit and have sundowners, watching life slow down as the light went out of the day. We would watch Aiden run around with wild abandon, exploring the sand and water and life he found within it. Special moments. I can almost still taste the salt from the spray off the ocean.

The one great lesson that I have taken from this whole experience has been to take the moments from my life and imprint them in my memory. These moments can be anything from the simplest things—a taste, a smell, and a view—to something more profound. My appreciation of these moments is so much more heightened than it ever was before. For this I am thankful. My life may certainly not be perfect, but boy, are there some perfect moments.

January 20

For some reason, while on holiday in South Africa I have decided that I wanted to actually make the trip to Baltimore to see Dr. Q in person for my next follow up. I can get my annual MRI done there and see him afterwards for an appointment. I can also spend the weekend in New York and visit my brother's best friend, my 'North American brother.' A win-win situation all round.

So I make the trip in the chill of January 2012 to the world-renowned Johns Hopkins Hospital in Baltimore. Flying over white snow-covered landscapes, I wonder what will await me.

What awaits me is a colloid cyst that has not really changed in size at $1.3 \times 1.2 \times 1.3$ cm. My neurological exam is normal. Dr. Q recommends that I definitely continue with the yearly MRIs and evaluations, and said that surgical intervention is not recommended at this point. My symptoms are being adequately managed by my current medication regime. On average, I get a migraine that requires my migraine medication every two months. Otherwise, ibuprofen seems to do the job.

I am very glad that I came. It is good to be able to meet him in person; somehow it puts things in perspective.

January 24

So, back home it is. Back to work, back to husband and son and work and life. All the reasons that I changed my work dynamics are working out. I am able to drop Aiden at school and collect him as well; I can participate in all the volunteer activities at school and do play dates in the afternoons as well.

Today in the doctor's waiting room I noticed an interesting pamphlet on 'Team in Training.' It is all about joining their Team in Training program to do a half or full marathon to support people with a variety of blood cancers through the Leukemia & Lymphoma Society of Canada.

This sounds like a great and worthwhile adventure for me to pursue and so I am going to do it—but only the walking half marathon, no running for me with an arthritic hip! Hoping I can do this —the farthest I have ever walked or run is ten kilometers, and now I will be doing double that at twenty-one kilometers. But they have a comprehensive training program and help you all the way through, including the fundraising part. So, I sign up for the BMO Vancouver Half Marathon 2012.

I start the training program and meet up with others each Sunday to start walking. In no time at all I find I am already at the ten-kilometer mark—it is really a great energizer and I am enjoying the challenge as well as the fundraising for such a worthy cause. This came at a really good time for me. Since having quit my job and started my own business, I have felt like something is missing. Not sure what it is, to be honest; I feel like I have everything I need. It might have been the transition from being in an office on a regular basis to being at home. It is a definite change of pace and rhythm, but I prefer it.

Training for the half marathon has now added another frame to my daily life, I walk each day and have another goal to achieve. I also find that by changing my focus and attention onto an area such as fundraising for individuals who have a life-threatening illness, I feel like I am making a difference. At the same time it is helping me move forward, in a positive way, from the last year and my own health challenges.

March 7

Before I know it, spring break is approaching and daylight saving is almost here. This is always a time of year I love: the spring bulbs are making their appearances known, their colors a changing visual display, the fresh green leaves starting to unfurl on the trees, life starting to come back into nature around us.

As a family, we have been investigating getting a puppy. Aiden is now almost six years old and he has been desperate for a dog. He is an only child and we figure it will be a good idea for him to have some company and have a pet to be attached to and love, as well as take responsibility for. We have been looking around and think we have found a match! We head out of town to look at the little white-with-black-mark Havanese pup. He looks like a puff of fur. Too sweet, you could just pick him up with one hand. His name is Bolt and he is nine weeks old. Aiden always wanted a dog just like the dog in the movie Bolt, so it seems like this match has already been made.

Two days before spring break, I meet a good friend of mine for a coffee and a walk on the sea wall before the next two weeks of school holidays begin. A beautiful day greets us as we walk, chatting. As we move towards the ocean, I feel as if my shin is aching. I have not turned or twisted my foot or ankle, but it feels like I've got a shin splint. I stop to massage it a bit and then we carry on. Afterwards, though, the top of my foot really starts to throb. "Not interested" I say to my foot. I think my legs may just be complaining, as I am now at around eighteen kilometers in my half-marathon training. I reckon it could be a cumulative thing. I will just ice my foot when I get home.

Unfortunately, the next day I wake up, jump out of bed ready to conquer the day, and hit the ground yelping. This is very painful indeed! Guess the ice and heat did not do the trick. My ankle is slightly swollen and I really cannot bear any weight on my foot. I resurrect my crutches from my bygone hip fracture out of the garage and get going on those.

No rest for me today—too much to do, including a visit to the doctor. She sends me off to the ER for an X-ray to ensure there is no fracture. They do a CT scan as well.

Before I even see the doctor I am confronted by a nurse wielding a very large needle and letting me know I am about to receive a tetanus shot. I flatly refuse, as I know how much those hurt and I am also needle phobic. I have not even seen a doctor yet but am getting an injection; how can that work? The doctor arrives. He examines my foot and sees there is no cut and hence no tetanus injection required. I heave a huge sigh of relief. The CT scan shows I have torn a ligament in my ankle and will be in an Aircast boot for four to six weeks. I will be on crutches until it heals. Great start to spring break. I did not just have my son joining me for two weeks, but also an Aircast boot, crutches, and one very sore foot. Oh well, this too shall pass. But after having raised over $1,400 for the Leukemia and Lymphoma Society, it seems my hopes of walking the half-marathon this May will have to be put on hold.

March 15

Our little pup has also arrived home. The bundle of fur prances around the garden like a cotton-wool ball, then passes out stone cold on the couch. Aiden thinks this is awesome.

And so, life with Bolt begins. He is very cute. Lots of work, but cute. I arrange puppy lessons and find a doggy daycare for when I have to go to a client meeting for the day. Doggy walks become part of our daily routine. Spring is here and summer is beckoning.

We are heading to Europe this summer, which is very exciting. Aiden and I are going to spend the first week in the United Kingdom visiting family and a dear friend of mine, then Marchand will join us and we will go to Florence, Italy and then to Siena and Sardinia. All in all, we will be gone four weeks.

Having a puppy now means finding a home for him while we are gone. Luckily enough, we find a home for him just down the road with a local dog-sitter, and she is great. So we are ready for our Tuscan adventure and for catching up with family and friends beforehand. Pasta, pizza and balsamic vinegar—here we come.

Five

SUMMER REPRIEVE

July 31

Summer has arrived in Vancouver. All the trees are full of green, the flowers are out, the colors are everywhere and people are walking around with smiles on their faces. One thing that I do love about the northern hemisphere is the very distinct changes between seasons. So dramatic. In the southern hemisphere, it is more like a blur between spring and summer, and then between fall and winter.

We are back from a wonderful family holiday in Europe. Such lovely sights and sounds and memories. We spent a fantastic week, just Aiden and I, in the United Kingdom seeing one of my best friends from South Africa with her gorgeous brood. In fact, the last little munchkin had only just arrived weeks before our arrival. Fun in the sun was had with all the kids running in the sunny garden stark naked, enjoying the joys of child hood.

We also spent time seeing family, which was special. Aiden had such a great time; his first question was when would he see his cousins again? Then onto Florence, Siena and Sardinia. Lots of sun for us all, in fact it was super hot. Aiden looked like a beach child, with a lovely tanned skin and bleached blond hair.

Now that we are back home it is a mixture of days spent with friends at the beach, summer camps and just relaxing. No running out the door to a scheduled agenda, but rather days out enjoying the best time of the year here in Vancouver. I cannot believe it is only the end of July and we still have the whole of August left before back to school.

Little did I know that the following month would become the most challenging of my life. Little did I know what was growing at a rapid rate inside my head.

I am still getting used to the ten-week summer holiday system here in Canada. As a child, we had at most twelve weeks holiday the whole year. But I cannot complain, since it allows us the freedom to enjoy the warm weather and summer activities.

My folks were also booked to come out for the next three weeks to spend time with us—we were so looking forward to seeing them. Unfortunately, Dad has such a painful back at the moment that long distance travel is a challenge. So they cancelled the trip; what a pity.

The strange thing is that Dad just called me just this morning. He said that he had been thinking over the past day about their trip cancellation and something inside him, a feeling, made him think they really needed to come to Vancouver. So, he had been back to the travel agent and rebooked their tickets for the twenty-fourth of August.

I have had that feeling only once in my life before. Sometimes for no reason in particular, your mind tells you this is just something you need to do.

Looking back months on, this decision of theirs would be our saving grace.

Hey, my medical alert bracelet arrived today. My husband and I discussed me getting one while we were in Europe, in case I ever had a seizure or became unconscious due to my cyst.

At the end of it all, I wore the bracelet for only just under one month. It was as if this play of life was going to happen regardless of anything I did.

Six

DOWNHILL:
THE SLIPPERY SLOPE

I REMEMBER THIS DAY AS BEGINNING THE LAST CHAPTER OF this whole saga. I sometimes feel like my health has been divided into the Harry Potter series of books. This is the last book. The finale, but not quite.

August 8

My body's waking up, my ears hear sounds of life around me. My eyelids rebel against the waking of the day. Open now! Hang on, the room is not still. It starts a familiar yet terrifying spin.

Oh no, not again. This time I feel my body lurching around as if on a wild sea, but I have not moved an inch. I squeeze my eyes shut in the vain hope that it will all go away - except it makes it worse. I open my eyes. After negotiating with my body, I slowly make my way to the washroom, stumbling over my own feet. Oh no, this is worse than the last time I had a vertigo attack.

I make it to the washroom just in time and am sick to my stomach. The toilet bowl and I become firm friends as I clutch on for dear life. The vertigo makes it presence known for what feels like an hour then releases its hold on me. I feel like an empty peanut shell; all my strength has gone and I am now just the leftover husk.

It is summer holidays; my son is at home for another six weeks and I am barely able to stand upright. Thank goodness for my husband, who is able to work at home and watch over him as I lie in bed, willing myself to recover and be 'back to normal.'

It is hard to describe the lethargy and physical exhaustion that comes after these vertigo attacks. Just lifting my arms off the bed feels like a weightlifting contest. On day two the room is not spinning but I am left with a mugginess, a fogginess that fills my brain and every fiber of my body. Climbing the stairs is a monumental effort, I have trained for a half-marathon before and this feels more challenging—seriously?

August 10

After two days of still feeling yuck, I am off to see my GP. She does a brief neurological examination and notices that I am struggling with my upward gaze. When she asks me to look up, I feel like my eyes are getting stuck at the top. How strange! I have not felt that before.

Given the colloid cyst and the fact that I am battling to look up and still suffering from the effects of my vertigo attack, my GP sends me to see a neurologist at the referral hospital, just to check everything out. She's a new neurologist to the practice; she has in fact just graduated, and is the locum for my usual neurologist. She does a thorough examination and says that I am most likely suffering from labyrinthitis or vestibular neuritis, which is causing my vertigo.

Her advice is to take my Serc medication (anti-vertigo medication) as required. With time, it should pass, but I am to come back if any other symptoms occur.

She does not say anything about the fact that my eyes feel stuck; she suggests it might be a subjective thing that I'm feeling, but that I could actually look upwards when she examined me.

Okay, that seems logical to me. Life goes on. So we have a lovely week with friends, out at the beach in the sun. The kids have been playing in the water, building their own rivers with stones and just enjoyed being kids. My vertigo has mostly gone and not made a debut performance, thank goodness. I just feel tired and off balance. Taking my Serc and that seems to help. I would never drive with Aiden if I felt unstable.

I was able to pop into the city today to see a dear friend of mine, an ex-work colleague, for coffee while Aiden was at soccer camp. My friend has just found out he has Hodgkin's lymphoma and has started treatment for it. I am so glad we got to touch base, as I have been worried about him and wanted to show my support. My nausea was overwhelming this morning, though, and I had to chomp down a huge muffin while we chatted, to keep from feeling ill. It reminded me of morning sickness.

Oh hang on...familiar feeling. After coffee I rushed to the pharmacy and grabbed a pregnancy test. This would be a true miracle if this happened, given everything I have been through in trying to actually have a baby in the past.

Not pregnant. Not sure how that makes me feel.

August 16

Today, we go off together for a mom-and-son date at the movies to see *Ice Age 3: Dawn of the Dinosaurs*. There is something magical about going to a kid's movie. Such excitement, yells of happiness when the movie starts and a continuous commentary from little people in the dark—just part of the setting! I never realized this until taking Aiden to his first movie show.

We had a fun time; so much fun that I think my head is maxed out. I can feel a migraine coming on. That crippling pain moves down my neck and then up over my head, behind my eyes. I decide to take an Axert quickly and hope it will prevent it from going any further. Summer is here, I am at home with Aiden and really don't want a migraine to spoil things.

August 17

Okay, so the Axert is doing very little to get rid of this ever-growing migraine. My eyes feel like they are going to explode out of their sockets. My neck is incredibly painful, I feel nauseous and the light is way too bright. I have been using cold packs, hot packs—anything to help relieve my head. The same on the medication front, a mixture of anything between Tylenol, Advil, and my usual migraine medicines...let me try sinus medication and sprays; maybe I have a sinus infection. Nothing is working. Hmmm. Might need some help here.

August 18

Off to my GP. This migraine is going nowhere—I want it out of here! I have to say at this point, that my GPs (a husband and wife team) have been amazing caregivers for us as a family since we arrived in Canada. I do feel they make the best decisions for us and have a great combination of both empathy and astute medical savvy. My GP has now prescribed a combination of Tylenol No. 3 and Advil to see if that will break through the migraine.

August 20

It is now day five on migraine watch. The migraine is still here and not budging. It is not insanely painful, but it just won't go away. My GP has advised that I must go to the ER the next day if it does not break and get them to look me over, as they may need to do further investigations or be more aggressive with the medications. Thank goodness we have a great student babysitter I found over the summer. She comes every so often to look after Aiden. I have used her quite a bit the past couple of days, as my migraine needs a dark and quiet room and not the bright sunlight and screams of childlike excitement emanating from the back yard.

August 22

Waking up on day seven, my migraine is as evident as it was on day one. Nothing has changed and none of the medications have touched it. I leave early for the ER, as I am desperate to get rid of this. I would also prefer to get them to check that this has nothing to do with my brain. Given it is now day seven, I think enough is enough.

I have never been a fan of the ER setting. It pulses with energy, both positive and negative, and is often full of people who are sick or about to be sick. I just feel sad for them all. The other side is the wait. Unless you are having a cardiac arrest or bleeding profusely from a visible source, get your book out and get ready to read and wait...for a long time. Such is the nature of the ER.

I hope since I have arrived early it will not be too chaotic. It is 7 am. I go through triage and tell them that I have a colloid cyst and have had a severe vertigo episode and now a migraine for seven days. My GP said to come to the ER for further investigation should it not resolve with the medication regime she gave me.

I wait for about two hours before I get to go through for examination. The ER doctor eventually comes to me, does a brief examination and gets an IV started for some migraine meds. I ask the doctor if they are going to do a CT scan. He looks quite confused as to why I would ask for a CT scan. I say, because of my colloid cyst. No reaction. Just confusion.

All right let's try a different tactic. "Because of my non-malignant brain tumor." Now that gets a reaction.

"You have a brain tumor?" he asks with big eyes.

"Yes, a colloid cyst in the third ventricle, it is on my chart".

"Do you have a neurosurgeon or neurologist I can contact?"

I give him the details. He is able to get hold of the neurologist, the same one I saw just under two weeks ago for my vertigo attack. The neurologist says there is no need for a CT scan or further imaging and that I must go back to my GP should the symptoms not resolve after giving me the IV migraine medications.

I have found in general that something about the words colloid cyst does not evoke an immediate response from some medical staff. I sometimes think that it is because they are not sure what it is. This is totally understandable. Medicine has fields of specialty because the human body is such a complex entity. So, when dealing with people who are not specialists in the field of neurology or neurosurgery, I tend to refer to my "non-malignant brain tumor in the third ventricle of my brain" instead of a colloid cyst. The response is completely different. Worlds apart. Black and white. That is one reason I also got my medical alert bracelet to state very clearly the medical history I had—colloid cyst of the third ventricle. This, at least, helps point an arrow in the right direction should it be needed. "It's over here! Look in here, in the brain."

Eventually, I leave the ER feeling quite dosed up on meds. My husband and son come to fetch me and I aim to sleep it off and feel a new person upon waking. Yes, I will be a new person ready to take on the rest of summer. I am lucky enough to be able to send Aiden to his best friend's house for a play date while I rest up in bed.

We arrive home and my husband is not convinced that the treatment I have received at the ER is up to standard. "Why did they not do a quick

CT scan? Seriously, just send Dr. Q a quick email to ask him what he thinks about your symptoms."

I agree that makes sense; a second opinion is never a bad thing. So the next morning, with my migraine still pounding despite the ER staff telling me it should be gone, I type out my email.

August 23

<u>*Email to Johns Hopkins*</u>

Dear Dr. Q,

I came to see you in January 2012 for monitoring of my colloid cyst. I had the MRI done at Johns Hopkins and then saw you for a consult afterwards.

I just have a quick question for you.

2 weeks ago, I had a vertigo attack with extreme nausea and vomiting. After the attack had finished (couple of hours), I just felt tired and still nauseous and dizzy. My doctor said I had vestibular neuritis and put me on Serc. Over the past 2 weeks, I still experience nausea all the time, dizziness and lack of balance. On Thursday last week, I developed a migraine worse than any migraine I have ever had. I tried Axert, Tylenol, sinus meds etc. My doctor changed me to Tylenol and ibuprofen, which helped for 1 day. She told me to go direct to the ER if nothing improved. So, yesterday I went to the ER and they gave me an IV migraine med, which helped for a short time (i.e. 12 hours).

I have woken up again this morning with a migraine and imbalance. The doctors yesterday said that these symptoms were nothing to do with my cyst. Should I just carry on and hope this stops by itself?

Well. Let's see what Dr. Q. says.

Within the hour, I get a response from my neurosurgeon in the United States, who has cc'd his physician's assistant to call me. I am always impressed with how prompt and professional they are. They really make me feel like I am in good hands and they care about me and my health. I never feel like I am just another patient, another number.

I just spoke to Jill, the physician assistant and she said that I really need to get an MRI done to rule out any hydrocephalus.

Now I must arrange for a private MRI again, but I know I will feel better if I can be sure that there is nothing strange going on. I have been to the neurologist, been to the ER and have no straight diagnosis or way forward. Time to hand over to my second opinion to be sure. My folks are also booked to arrive from South Africa on Friday afternoon, so it's best to get this all out the way before they arrive. I am sure it will all work out just fine.

Seven

QUICKSAND

August 24

It's now Friday. I have told my folks that I have had vertigo and now a migraine, so they know that I am not feeling one hundred percent. I have just text messaged them to let them know that I have organized someone to fetch them from the airport, as their flight arrives at the exact time that I have been able to schedule an MRI.

I lie waiting for my MRI at the private clinic on the other side of town. Not quite sure what to feel. I know Mom and Dad are by now in the car I have organized and on their way to our house. I cannot wait to see them. I cannot wait to get this MRI over and find out what is going on. I hope it is nothing. I am honestly just tired of feeling tired and not knowing what is going on. My migraine still lingers in the background. It has been around for over nine days like a dark cloud in the sky, and I am waiting for it to either rain or disappear over the horizon.

After I get my MRI CD, with no written report yet, I head on home. It is so wonderful to see my folks—nothing like a hug from Mom and

Dad to make you feel good. We have a lovely weekend catching up, enjoying the good weather. I sleep and try to get myself back on track. Amazingly, my migraine finally breaks on Sunday, day eleven. What a relief! It must have been a combination of all the medications that were thrown at it. I still feel very tired and off balance but without the migraine, things must be getting better, right? I am sure the MRI report will show nothing.

August 27

It is now Monday morning. My legs feel so tired, I feel like I am dragging lead around and I keep on bumping into things. My head feels thick and muggy even though my migraine has broken. I feel like I have to search through the folds of my brain when I need to think about saying something. Maybe I overdid it yesterday when we had our friends over to celebrate my folks being in town?

I have not yet received my report from the MRI. I suppose my body is now in recovery mode, although this brain and body fog I am now feeling is quite weird. I think I may need to see the GP again.

It is mid-Monday morning when my email buzzes: you have mail! It is my MRI report. I take a deep breath and open the report.

The key finding of hydrocephalus jumps straight out at me. I pause. I am not really sure what I feel at this moment. I feel glad they have found there is a reason for my insane and unforgiving migraine and I suppose also for the way my body and brain is feeling now. I suddenly feel scared, as I think I know what the answer is without asking: brain surgery.

I also feel completely lost, as my neurosurgeon is across the continent, in another country. Given what has happened over the past year, and especially in the last week, my faith in my referral hospital is rock-bottom low. What would have happened if we had not gone this route ourselves? The initial MRI still needs to be compared to the one done twelve months back, so I wait for an updated MRI report. In the meantime, I call Marchand and email him the report. Thank goodness he pushed me to have this MRI done.

MRI report

There is a lesion at the level of the foreman of Monro, which presumed represents a colloid cyst. There does appear to be some distension of the lateral ventricles consistent with hydrocephalus and there is transependymal flow. Comparison with the patient's previous exams is required to determine if there is significant interval change to explain the patient's acute symptoms. Once the imaging becomes available for review an addendum report can be issued.

Johns Hopkins has asked that I upload my MRI images to their server so they can have a look at them. You have to love technology—there is no need for me to mail the CD to them and wait another couple of days for their input. I upload the MRI images and the first report that I have just received to Johns Hopkins and they have them in a matter of minutes.

Email to Johns Hopkins

MRI almost uploaded for you to view (at 71% upload!).

Thanks so much. I have attached the radiology report that I received 10 minutes ago. They are going to compare the MRI done Friday with my previous one and resend the report as well. I will be interested to hear your comments on the hydro. I also noticed he did not comment on the size of the cyst so I have asked them to do so.

My migraine broke on Sunday after having it for over 11 days. I am still very dizzy, nauseated and my balance is off. So hoping the headache stays away—quite bizarre really.

Your advice is greatly appreciated!

Claire

I hear back immediately after the images have been uploaded. Dr. Q has reviewed the MRI and wants to talk to me about what this means later in the day, once he is out of surgery.

I walk up the stairs to tell my parents the latest results. My legs are feeling even heavier than they were this morning. How do you tell your parents that your brain is swelling and you will most likely need brain surgery? I knew they were concerned about this whole episode. I tell them we will wait to speak to Dr. Q later before jumping the gun regarding the next steps. They both give me a huge hug and let me know that they will help out in any way possible but I can see this news is hard for them to bear. I know that once I drag my heavy legs out the door and back to my bed that their brave faces may fall away.

Exhausted, I sleep the day away, and when I wake up I wait anxiously for Dr. Q to call me.

I receive the revised MRI report, now that they have compared it against the previous one. The results definitely show the cyst has grown, almost fifty percent in six months. No wonder I feel so horrific. My cerebrospinal fluid (CSF) is blocked at the foreman of Monro, as my cyst has now grown big enough to cause an obstruction.

Impression: The mass identified at the level of the foreman of Monro demonstrates significant interval increase in size and changed in signal characteristics. The provided history states the patient has a known colloid cyst. Rapid enlargement in size and signal changes identified in this study can be seen with rapidly enlarging colloid cyst related to increased water content. Given the developing hydrocephalus and the patient's symptoms, an urgent neurosurgical consultation is warranted.

The lesion presently measures 1.8 cm anteroposterior, 1.9 cm height and 1.9 cm width. Almost 2 centimeters. My previous MRI in January this year, just six months ago, showed the cyst at 1.3 by 1.2 by 1.3 cm.

That is quite an increase in six months, given I have had this cyst my whole life. I suppose when it decides it is going to grow, it grows.

I now have what is called obstructive hydrocephalus, where the normal drainage of spinal fluid out of the brain's ventricles is blocked and the resulting pressure buildup can cause headaches, nausea, blurred vision, double vision or, in severe cases, even loss of consciousness.[11]

When Dr. Q calls he tells me in no uncertain terms that the time has come to get the cyst out. It is obstructing my CSF flow and hydrocephalus is the result. It needs to come out now. Given my past history with the neurosurgical team at Johns Hopkins, my confidence in Dr. Q and my lack of confidence in my referral hospital and specialist medical staff, we ask for a cost estimate for having the surgery in the United States.

Funny, when we get the cost estimate back, it is lower than the one I got from UCLA a while back—we feel like we are getting a discount! The cost is still astronomical. We are lucky we can afford to do this. It will still not be petty cash and holidays will be on hold for quite a while, but when you are looking at life and potential death, the money doesn't matter.

We agree to go ahead with the surgery in the United States and start madly searching for flights, hotels and everything else that goes with having brain surgery. I am feeling okay. I am just so tired and my body is so heavy. I think the adrenalin surge that is coursing through my body now is what is keeping me standing and able to keep going, to a certain extent.

11 http://www.hopkinsmedicine.org/neurology_neurosurgery/specialty_areas/headache/conditions/obstructive_hydrocephalus.html

August 28

The next twenty-four hours are a blur for me. My dad decides to stay in Vancouver as he is struggling daily with a back condition and travel is a big challenge. He will also look after our dog and house, so it works out for the best. Mom will come with to look after Aiden. So my folks have been in Vancouver for only five days and now we are about to embark on our trip to Baltimore.

At this point things start to take a turn for the worse for me. I feel absolutely sapped of any energy, my mind feels like it is turning to mush and I feel my memory slowing. I feel like it is more of an effort to talk now, almost like I am slurring my words. I am exhausted, mentally and physically. My husband writes to the team at Johns Hopkins to inform them of the change in my condition. They want me there as soon as possible. Surgery is scheduled for four days away: Friday, August 31.

Marchand's email to Johns Hopkins says:

Claire is getting progressively more tired each day—for the last week or so she has needed to rest (sleep) in the afternoon but she now needs to start resting at 11h00 (after 8 hours sleep during the night). Physically she is also becoming weaker—less stable (lack of coordination) and less able to feel her legs. Her short-term memory is also being impacted (not recalling incidents / actions that happened shortly beforehand) and she is routinely using the incorrect words. Not sure if this indicates a need for more urgent treatment but suffice to say it is troubling to watch.

Are there any symptoms I need to be aware of that may indicate a need to take her to the ER in the interim?

Given my prior history, I leave my medical records in a big red folder at the door with a note as to which hospitals to take me to and which not to if need be. I also leave Dr. Q's phone number and my GP's number on the front. I let my folks know that if I go unconscious or have a seizure and they need to call an ambulance, here are my files and requests. Not a great discussion to have with one's parents. I can see the concern in my parent's eyes well up in the unshed tears and know that behind the door of their room, their true feelings about this situation are being unleashed.

I cannot imagine what this must feel like for my husband. He is watching me deteriorate before his eyes and knows I am going to have brain surgery. But first we have to fly across the country and into the United States, before I am safely delivered into the hands of my neurosurgeon.

In my moments of clarity I move around, packing and sending emails to Aiden's school, our friends and one to my dear dad with all the details for the house while we are away. Marchand and I organize accommodation, flights and everything else. Baltimore is an amazing city with regards to accommodation. Given its large number of very prominent and internationally-renowned hospitals and medical centers, you can get patient discounts at most hotels. This allows us to book into a really nice hotel that I know will look after Mom and Aiden while Marchand and I are engaged in other things, such as brain surgery.

August 29

Hi everyone,

I am sending a 'group' email as we are in a rush today! If you are not aware, I am heading off to Johns Hopkins (Baltimore) for brain surgery. We just got confirmation for Friday surgery this morning. So action stations! My colloid cyst has increased dramatically in size over the past while and I have been unwell for the past 2-3 weeks. The end result is they need to take the cyst out immediately as I have hydrocephalus which needs to be treated ASAP. The op will take about 4 hours and I will be in hospital for 3-4 days afterwards but have to remain in Baltimore for 5 days after that to ensure everything is good.

Lots of love

Claire

I remember my dear dad coming into my room as I was resting after the chaos of the morning. He had tears in his eyes as he wished me all the best and said he would be thinking of me all the time. This must be a terribly hard thing to do, wave your daughter off on a flight to another country where she is about to undergo brain surgery.

After saying goodbye to my dear Dad, with tears in my eyes and fatigue in my body, we head off to the airport. On the way we stop at my husband's office to get the Power of Attorney he has organized for my surgery. As I sign it, the reality of the situation sinks in a little deeper. This step might be morbid, but it is important.

My wheelchair arrives as we check in for our flight. I can barely walk a few steps; my legs are too heavy, weak and numb. After the mammoth walk from the cab drop-off area to the check-in counter —a distance of maybe twenty meters—I am quite happy to be seated in the wheel-chair. This is all such a blur to me. As we wait to board our plane, my GP calls me to ask if my neurosurgeon has said anything about the risk of flying while having hydrocephalus. I quickly email Dr. Q and he reassures me that the risk is minimal and I can get on the plane.

My mom and I sit together while Aiden and Marchand sit at the back of the plane—we booked in such a hurry that we could not even get four seats together; in fact we had to beg to get me to be able to sit next to my mom. We explained that my son had to have someone with him and I too had to have someone with me, given my current health situation.

We are right at the front of economy class and I am desperate for the washroom. Looking back to the economy class washroom at the back of the plane, I know it is too far for me to walk. I go to the business class washroom a couple of rows ahead. Relief. Until I get a talking-to by the air hostess who rudely informs me that I am not allowed to come here, and that she has a full business class. I am too tired to argue with her or let her know that I physically cannot make it to the back of the plane. So the tears just fall down my face.

We are half way to Baltimore now. Overnight in Toronto and staying in an airport hotel for five hours, then up and out to catch our next plane. I remember my husband stroking my hair while I was falling asleep. I later asked him why he did that and he said he was scared that I was going to stroke out beside him.

August 30

Arriving in Baltimore is a relief; we are at least in the right city and closer to sorting me out and getting the medical attention I need. The plane was a bit cold on the way down from Toronto so I had wrapped myself up in the Wall Street Journal that was handed out by the steward—quite a laugh, looking back! We check my mom and Aiden into the hotel then give them a hug good bye and take a cab straight to the hospital.

I don't even remember being emotional about it—I felt like I was exist-ing in a cloud up in the sky, looking down on and not part of what was happening. My brain was swelling.

At the hospital, the nursing staff settles me into my room on the neu-rosurgical floor. They put an IV in and I am immediately off to have my stereotactic MRI, which they will use tomorrow in the surgery. Stereotactic brain surgery is where MRI images are used to help guide the surgeon to the exact location of the tumor.

I am starving, since I only ate a muffin for breakfast and it is now lunchtime. "Sorry, no food for you," they tell me. "You are now nil per mouth in case anything changes and you require emergency surgery." So that Philly steak sandwich they were telling me about when I arrived may need to wait! Aagh.

At the time I had not thought about even asking how they were going to get my cyst out and to this day I don't remember if they even told me. All I knew was it had to come out. No options here. But just for the notes, I had an endoscopic craniotomy.

So I head off to MRI and come out with lovely circular stickers on my face, encircled by permanent marker. These were used in the MRI to help with the mapping and will also be used tomorrow in the surgery. So they will stay on my face overnight. I look a sight but hey, that is the last thing on my mind right now. I take a video on my iPhone for Aiden, as I will not see him before my surgery tomorrow. I show him my cool stickers and tell him that Mommy is doing all right and that I love him lots. No doubt he would tell me I look like I have bullet holes in my face.

The rest of the afternoon is spent having all other pre-op testing done such as chest X-rays as I am asthmatic, blood tests for blood typing and general blood analysis and anything else they need done in preparation. I feel like I am in very capable hands.

Eight

THE CUTTING EDGE

I FINALLY GET TO SEE THE 'MAN OF THE MOMENT.' DR. Q AR-
rives to chat to me. In the past few hours I have already seen his
resident doctors several times. He arrives with a great smile and tells
me he is so happy to see me here and knows that I am in the right
place, and that everyone is going to take good care of me. I feel relieved. He does a quick medical exam and notices that I am getting
more lethargic and my words are slowing.

"How long has she been like this?" he asks.

I tell him I have been feeling more and more tired over the past hour
or so.

"Let's move her to ICU just in case we need to place an external
ventricular drain in overnight." He explains that in the ICU
(Intensive Care Unit), they can keep a more critical eye on me in
case my brain swelling gets out of control and if they need to place
an external ventricular drain.

So off we go. They ask for my husband's cell number so they can call
him and let him know of the change in situation. Poor Marchand,

getting a call to say "By the way, don't worry but we are just moving your wife to ICU as she is declining."

"I will see you for 7 am surgery tomorrow," Dr. Q says as he leaves. "You will be fine, and these good doctors and nurses will keep a good eye on you so I can get this sorted out."

What is it really like in ICU? I have been in ICU many times, as a visitor a few times to see sick friends, as a health care professional, many times. As a patient—never. At Johns Hopkins, in the Neurosciences Critical Care Unit, each patient has an individual room that is glassed in facing onto a central nursing station. Inside, a myriad of monitors are strapped onto your body. There is no longer silence. You can hear nurses outside the room, bleeps and noises from all the machines, both in your own room and outside. I have my IV in, blood pressure cuff on, electrodes on that monitor my heart rate, and pulse oximeter that monitors my oxygen saturation.

I doze on and off in the haze of the ICU until Marchand comes back early evening to visit. I can see he is anxious. The next time I wake it is 2 am and the clock seems to be moving so slowly. My nurse, Donna, tells me that Marchand went back to the hotel around 1 am and will be back at 6 am to see me before my 7 am surgery.

Donna and I chat on and off through the night as she comes in every hour to check my vitals and neurological status. All I can hear is the continuous bleeping of the machines around me. I suddenly realize that I have not really said goodbye to my Mom or Aiden and will not see them again before my surgery. This hits home. I ask Donna to help me get my pen and paper out of my bag. I will write a short note to Aiden and one to my folks, one to Marchand and one to my brother.

Wow, what to write? They say at the end of it all, you see your life flash before you. Well, I am most certainly not at the end but I want to ensure that they know just how much they mean to me and how much

I love them, in case something goes wrong and I cannot tell them myself. This is bringing tears to my eyes. I do wish I could give Aiden a hug and kiss before the surgery. I am trying to remember what I said to him and my mom before saying goodbye at the hotel before we went to the hospital, but my brain is too sore, it is too tired, and it feels too swollen. Well, my notes will say how I feel. I write them and feel much better. I close my eyes and fall asleep to the noises of the ICU. My notes lie waiting on the table beside my bed.

August 31

It's 6 am and my support rock arrives, my husband. I am not sure if he even got any sleep. The ICU, the heart of the hospital, has been action stations since about 4:30 am, as it normally is. Getting people ready for surgery, giving patients their meds before doctors' rounds. The ICU is never silent.

My tummy grumbles. I am very hungry, as the last thing I ate was at this time yesterday morning. I am looking forward to my first meal already. I hope the hospital does not live up the normal reputation of 'hospital food'! I have completely forgotten any sense of what I look like or when I last brushed my teeth or my hair or washed my face. I honestly don't care. My brain is focused on a much bigger picture. I feel so incredibly tired and out of it, like I am in a constant fog. Just lifting my arms is an effort.

It's now time. Off we go to the operating room (OR) and everyone in the ICU says bye, good luck and see you later! Wish it were this easy. In the OR admission area a steady stream of people come and poke and prod me, take vitals, I sign forms, Marchand signs forms, they sign in black permanent marker on my right forehead to confirm this is the approach to be used. This would make for a great Facebook photo: me plastered with the stereotactic MRI stickers all over my face and black permanent marker on my forehead. But as I said, vanity at this stage is really not my key concern.

I see Dr. Q before he goes to get some breakfast and his positive, energetic manner reassures me that this is all going to be okay. I feel calm. He is one of those people who exude a sense of positivity and compassion for his patients and their families. Having worked over the years with many specialists across many medical disciplines, I know that his combination of skill and empathy are unusual. You could hug him.

The anesthesiologist and her nurses come and chat. "Please", I tell them, "give me anything to help with the post-op nausea, as my body has a habit from previous experience of rebelling and reacting badly when I wake up."

They ask me if there is anything else I need before going under.

"Please, can someone just hold my hand?"

It is time to go to the operating room. I say goodbye to Marchand, I tell him I love him and gulp down my tears. It is now all so very real. I am not scared, just sad. Wheeling down the cold hall of the OR corridor, I know Marchand is watching me. I already miss him, and I love him so much. I cannot imagine what it feels like to be in his shoes at this moment. He is going to stay in the 'family' room and wait.

The operating room buzzes with activity; scrub nurses and other people move around with trays in their hands. I am not going to be my usual curious self. Too many sterile trays with too many things inside that I don't really want to see.

I transfer from my warm bed to the colder operating table and stare up into the bright lights. The medical staff start looking at my veins and strapping all the monitors onto my body—as if there was space for any more. I can feel the tears coming. I feel so very vulnerable. My life is literally in someone else's hands.

They wrap me in several warm toasty blankets to stave off the cold of the operating room and bustle around me like busy bees for what feels like five or ten minutes. The anesthetic nurses I spoke to in the OR admission area are there, and it is comforting to see a set of familiar eyes behind the masks. They chat to me as if we are out having a cup of coffee.

I have been an observer in many operations over my career and it is always a strange thing to hear people talk about their day and carry on normally while performing surgery. But for these people, it is their everyday lives, so why not? The last thing I remember is the kind eyes of the anesthetic nurse as he said, "it's time now." He held my hand, and so did the other nurse. I felt calm, then the prickle of the general anesthetic and the strange taste in my mouth and...

Nine

LIGHT DAWNS

August 31 (Day 1 post surgery)

<u>*Email to family and friends*</u>

Hi everyone,

Claire is out of surgery and according to the doctor it went well—although cyst much bigger than expected. She is in recovery but initial neurological exam looks good—follows instructions etc.

Will probably update again tomorrow, as today will very much be a recovery day for Claire.

Thank you for your good wishes and thoughts, it is highly appreciated

Marchand and Aiden

<u>*Excerpt from Operative Report (August 31)*</u>

Endoscopic resection to the right Kocher's point for the resection of a colloid cyst in the foramen of Munro. A #22 modifier for the increased level of complexity by at least 50% given the size of the tumor, the location of the tumor, and the fact it was surrounded by several veins going into the venous angle including the septal vein as well as the thalamostriate, and the carotid vein. All this increased the level of complexity as well as the time it took to resect the tumor that was all infiltrated with the foramen of Monro.

The first thing I remember is opening my eyes and seeing a very blurred figure standing in the door of my ICU room. I knew immediately it was my husband, as I knew his frame, the way he stood, and could vaguely see his familiar shirt. I had a second to acknowledge seeing him before the massive wave of nausea hit me. I dry heaved while the nurses ran around with syringes filled with anti-nausea medications, hoping to find one that would give me relief.

Coming out of general anesthesia is always a bizarre experience for me. You are stuck between the worlds of real and unreal and feel like you are trying to swim up to the surface, only to get pushed under again. I feel like my body is on fire, my limbs feel prickly and I ask the nurse in my slurred speech: "Have I had a stroke? " I could not lift my limbs.

"Not at all, you are good, you did so well. Look, lift your leg."

Lo and behold my leg rises off the bed. I close my eyes again.

My husband told me later that when I started coming around post-op and I was so confused and slurring, he thought I had had a stroke or brain damage. I cannot imagine being in his shoes, looking into my ICU room and seeing my spouse, my life partner, in this situation. I thought that all the words I was trying to say were vaguely identifiable but my husband said that I sounded like a cow mooing. Well, that was a first! We all had a good giggle about that well after my recovery.

My nurse Tatiana is a gem and she helps me through those first hours. It seems she is always by my side.

At this point I am firmly attached to my bed. I have my IV line, my arterial line (used to monitor blood pressure real-time and to obtain blood samples for arterial blood gas measurements and other such interesting things), my catheter, my pulse oxymeter, my external ventricular drain out my head (allowing drainage of cerebrospinal fluid), calf cuffs on my legs (to prevent clots) hissing on and off, and heart monitors. I am literally held hostage in bed by these contraptions.

I don't remember much of that first day post surgery apart from coming around from the anesthetic and then sinking back into a welcome slumber. I remember the neurosurgical resident who helped Dr. Q with my surgery coming to see me and check on my ventricular drain—they 'upped' the drainage, which apparently could increase the nausea but was necessary. I would only realize in the next day or so that I had a drain sticking out my head! I remember being so relieved to see my husband. Just knowing he was there was my link to reality and a sense that I had gotten through; everything was now going to be okay.

According to my husband, the surgery went well. I had a craniotomy. This is where they removed part of the bone of my skull in order to get to my brain. The operation was then performed using endoscopic equipment. The operation was more complicated than originally thought, as some of the veins were wrapped around the cyst and it took longer to resect as a result. It was good timing that the cyst was removed—not just because of the hydrocephalus, but also because the veins around the cyst were taking a lot of pressure from the growing cyst. Just like a balloon, veins can take only so much pressure before they burst. Timing is everything.

Hi

Thank you for your emails—Claire had a good night (other than being wakened up every hour for a neurological exam)—her neurological exams are all normal and her ICP (intracranial pressure) so far is within the normal range. She will be in ICU for 2 more days to assess the need (or not) for a shunt.

Regards

Marchand and Aiden

September 1 (Day 2)

I wake up during my second night in ICU. Amidst the bleeps and sounds around me, everything else is quiet. I take a moment to take it all in. I am immensely thankful in that moment, grateful that I am there and everything has worked out well, that I was intact and fully functional (albeit strapped to my bed). I had a non-malignant brain tumor that had now been removed, and once I was recovered, that would be it, I hoped. In that silent hour by myself, I count my blessings.

The next day passes in a blur with doctor's visits and nurse's check ups. The routine neurological exam every couple of hours becomes a predictable part of the day. I still cannot fathom why they ask you what the date is as part of the neuro exam. Even when I am operating at my best capacity, ask me the date and I will look at you blankly. I will know what day it is, but not necessarily win gold on the exact date. So I learn to glance up at the board in my room, which shows the date. At least my cognitive abilities are intact!

It is strange, but I do not feel an immense amount of pain after the surgery. My head aches but not like I was expecting it to. They say that the brain does not have any pain receptors and hence does not feel the pain of having been operated on—that is a blessing. The parts that ache in my body are my arms, from all the IVs and the arterial line—that hurt the most, and I am developing a lovely deep blue purple bruise all along my arm. My IV seems to clog up a lot so they keep on having to find new sites. My arms feel riddled with holes.

My first bite of food is breakfast the day after my surgery. The oats porridge was the best I have ever had. In the hospital, food becomes a great event in your day as you choose your menu and then await the food's arrival. The clanking of the food carts down the hall brings on great excitement. I have a good appetite despite being just out of brain surgery.

I did not realize at that time that the dexamethasone[12] that I was being given daily by IV was fuelling a voracious appetite that would be around for a lot longer than I would have anticipated.

I think I must look like a robot of sorts. My head is swathed in a large bandage, I have a drain coming out my head, drips out of and into my arms and bleeping from the heart rate monitors on my chest and the cuffs on my legs that inflate and deflate on a regular basis. It's like something out of a science fiction novel. Aiden is not allowed to come into ICU and it is probably better, as I am not quite sure how he will react to seeing me looking like this.

Day by day, I get released from some of the 'entrapments' of my ICU bed. First the arterial line. It is a line they insert straight into your artery once you are under general anesthetic, in order to have direct access to your bloodstream. I did not realize how this would bruise and be so sore afterwards. Then the catheter—oh bliss. What a great feeling. Then the brain drain. Hope they did not take too much out the head—Marchand jokes with me, hoping they put an extra hard drive into my head when I was under—take something out, put something back in?

12 Dexamethasone: steroid used post brain surgery to decrease inflammation/swelling in the brain: http://www.nlm.nih.gov/medlineplus/druginfo/meds/a682792.html

September 2 (Day 3)

<u>Email to family and friends</u>

Claire had a follow up MRI and the doctors are happy with the out-come. She is doing well but tired (one of the main side effects of brain surgery) and the narcotics do their bit as well. Will probably stay in ICU for one more day then on to the ward.

Regards

Marchand and Aiden

My mom and Marchand have been alternating between looking after Aiden and me. They are my superstars. Aiden is having a great time, apparently: swimming at the hotel, eating cool food and building LEGO. What more could a six-year-old want? I get to see my Mom, and I can sense she is quite taken aback by my appearance. I am now developing a nice bruise under my right eye, and definitely look like I have taken a right hook. Apparently a bruised eye can occur post brain surgery. Well, I suppose I have been in the boxing ring with my tumor, but I won. Regardless, it was lovely to have her sit next to my bed even as I slept, and to know she was there watching over me.

I have not yet looked in the mirror. All I have seen is a short video I taped for Aiden to say hi to him. I have color back in my face now and still have permanent marker lines peeking out underneath my turbaned head. I have not even done my normal 'beauty routine' for the past three days. Lucky for my teeth, the nurses have ensured that is part of the routine!

"Okay, let's get you out of bed now," says my nurse.

"Seriously...now?" I ask.

He nods. I've got to get this body mobile and walking, it seems, is the first mode of transport. This certainly highlights the marvels of modern medicine; I am two days post brain surgery and about to embark on my first walk around the ICU.

They help me to sit upright on the edge of the bed and I feel like I imagine Neil Armstrong must have felt when he was about to step onto the moon. One small step for man, one giant leap for mankind. My legs feel weak but with the help of my hubbie and Guy, the ICU nurse, I manage a small loop around the ICU with the biggest smile on my face—this just makes things feel so good. My legs tire quickly and it's back to bed.

"We need to get you up and moving a couple of times a day," Guy says.

"Okay" I say, feeling like I am in training again for a half marathon.

Today Aiden comes to visit. Because he is not allowed in the ICU, I take the opportunity to use my walking time and walk just outside of the ICU to be with him. I will not forget the look on his face.

"You are not my mommy!" he says, as I walk slowly towards him. He jumps towards Marchand, who picks him up. I tell him I love him lots and will see him soon, and go straight back into the ICU before I traumatize him anymore.

Kids are amazingly resilient. They also react to change and situations such as ours in very different ways. Here was Aiden who had seen his Mom deteriorate from 'Mom in the super-woman cape' to Mom lying in bed, stumbling and not being able to look after him or herself, to Mom travelling to another country for emergency surgery and now full of drips and needles with her head in a bandage. For everything he went through at his age, he was remarkable. Yes, he still behaved like a normal six-year-old with the ups and downs and no's and everything else. But, as long as we were open about what was happening, he took it on board and carried on as if he were on holiday. However, I think the reality of this situation now in front of him was a bit too much.

Marchand became even more 'his world' than before. This hurt like hell but I understood it and knew that it would pass and time would heal it. In fact, when we called Aiden from the hospital for me to say hi, he briefly said hi to me and then wanted to immediately talk to Marchand and ask him when he was coming back to the hotel.

The word courage comes to mind when I think of my husband in particular. The definition of courage is: *Strength in the face of pain or grief.* Somehow he holds it together for us all. At the same time, I am acutely aware that this ongoing courage is tiring for him. Once we are home, it will be important for him to have some down time, time where he does not have to hold it together for everyone else.

As the day progresses, small things mean a big deal. Having my arterial line taken out, the monitors taken off my chest, my catheter out, drain removed from my head, bandage off my head, being able to walk a couple of steps unaided down the corridor. Small steps for mankind but big steps, in fact giant leaps, for me.

The physiotherapist in the unit assesses me to see how my progress is going. Her role is to ensure I am able to mobilize, get around safely and am functionally on track and to assess if I need any rehabilitation during my recovery. She goes over all the necessary support structures I will need at home and what I should be focusing on during my acute recovery.

I also see an occupational therapist, whose assessment is slightly different from that of the physiotherapist. She focuses more on how this surgery and the recovery may impact my day-to-day life, and how to work on conserving my energy. She looks at everything from "can I reach down to put on my own socks," to "can I reach over the table to find my pen." All the small things that one would not normally think of, but that can make a difference once you get home from hospital. She gave some solid advice on taking it slow and easy once we left the hospital and for example, not walking up and down the stairs at home all the time. This would sap my energy. Small steps, to allow me to be able to take those big steps in a shorter time frame!

September 3 (Day 4)

<u>*Email to family and friends*</u>

The brain drain tube was removed yesterday and no additional plumbing is required—first hair wash and bath (the bed variety) this morning and Claire went for a stroll yesterday morning—bit wobbly, but expected after being in bed for four days and having had brain surgery. Will most likely move to the neuro ward today from ICU. With luck Claire will write the next update

Marchand and Aiden

My first hair wash was fabulous! There is something about having your hair dreadlocked with antiseptic, caked blood and goop that does not leave you feeling your best. Forget having just had brain surgery. My vanity is now long gone and I am not worried about it at all, but after my hair is washed and dry I feel restored, and as if I could grace the cover of a magazine. Thank you, Nurse Guy, for my wonderful hair wash; I am now ready for anything!

I have been able to read a bit of a magazine. Not sure I could handle a massive novel, as that would indeed be a brain overload. Marchand has brought his laptop in and I have even read a few emails people have sent in, so I know my brain is functioning, which is good news. I have even switched on my phone and am going to connect, as one does in this day and age, with my friends all over the world using Facebook. Being from a marketing background, I do see the use of social media, although I'm not obsessed with it.

<u>*Facebook post: September 3*</u>

"What's on my mind," asks FB. Great question: lying in my neurosurgical ICU bed post op 3 days from removal of colloid cyst (non-malignant brain tumor) and thanking my lucky stars, my family (hubbie) and friends and amazing staff at Johns Hopkins for everything they have done to

get me to this stage. So what's on my mind...I am grateful for so much today I cannot get around to writing them down ☺"

September 4 (Day 5)

I have now been in the neuro ICU for five days now. I have had my hair washed, a glorious experience, and am free of any contraptions that could bind me to the bed or to the ICU. The staff have all been amazing. I am blessed to have been in this ICU and hospital where they have nursed me back to being able to leave only five days after brain surgery.

I am discharged directly from the ICU in my wheelchair. I leave with a bag full of medications and a list of instructions of what to take and when to take it. Thank goodness Marchand will be in charge of my medications, as I would not have a clue and would land up over- or under-medicating myself.

Driving back to the hotel I look out the window, wondering if things will feel different. I still feel weak, numb and 'out of my body,' but I know this too shall pass. Being back in the hotel room, seeing my mom and Aiden, feels like the best medicine I could ever ask for. We have to stay in town for another five days until I see Dr. Q again, and then we can go back to Canada. Back home.

Facebook post

September 4: All good, out of ICU and at hotel! Roll on proper bath and revived hair do ☺ feeling wobbly, sore head but relieved to have made it to the US for the op! Thx for everyone's concerns and kind wishes....Lots of love Claire

September 5 (Day 6)

Email to family and friends

Light Dawns

Claire was released from hospital yesterday afternoon and is recuperating at the hotel. We will be in Baltimore until next week, seeing surgeon on Monday for removal of stitches and follow up. Going well but still very tired.

Marchand and Aiden

I sink into my first proper bath filled with bubbles and feel the memories of the hospital melt away. I wash my body with the decadent L'Occitane soap provided by the hotel and the smell fills my senses.

My day consists of lots of sleep and just lying down, a medication regime like the military, and short walks to keep my body mobile in between the intense sleep. Between taking my dexamethasone (steroid), Tylenol (for pain), Zofran (for nausea and vomiting), Keppra (anti-seizure), Colace and Senna (to prevent constipation), PROTONIX (antacids) and waking at odd hours to take all these medications (bless my husband who sets his alarm every three hours, including during the night, to give them to me), the time passes.

Facebook post

Day 6 post op...Tired but happy to be out of hospital. Doc appointment next Wednesday so hoping to be home for the weekend!

Our schedules revolve around my sleep, waking to eat and take medications and then spending some time with my mom, Marchand and Aiden. I cannot believe how much I am sleeping. I wake up only to go to sleep again. I feel like everything is in slow motion. My body is so slow, every movement I make is slow, my thoughts seem slow, almost like through mud, but everything is working so I am pleased. At night, we walk slowly to a nearby restaurant for early dinner. It is good to be out and feel my body moving again and being part of the human race. Baltimore has some amazing food and it is nice that we get to enjoy some of the sights and sounds while we are here. I am amazed that I am able to actually have dinner out five days after having had brain surgery. Modern medicine is quite amazing. But then again we do have to eat! And for my mom, Marchand and Aiden, they have been here for almost two weeks, so going out to dinner is a nice change of scenery for them.

September 7

It is now day four out of hospital and I am finishing off some of my meds, including dexamethasone. I am still on the anti-seizure medication and will be for a while longer. Yippee, I no longer feel like an infant having to be woken every three hours to be fed! The boys go out to local museums or my mom takes Aiden swimming, but there is always someone with me in the room. The clocks tick on my recovery and we get closer to being able to go home. We are just waiting for the post-op visit to my neurosurgeon on Wednesday to get stitches removed and to get the A-okay to fly home.

September 9

Day six post hospital and I wake up with that familiar feeling of a blinding headache starting, but this time it is right across my forehead, like a metal bar has wacked me on the head. After taking various medications to try and relieve it, there is no progress. We phone Johns Hopkins who suggests taking some of the oxycodone I have from my time in hospital, which I do, but still no relief. Eventually, Dr. Q tells me to come to the ER to get a CT scan to make sure everything is okay post surgery. I feel nauseous as well.

I cling to Marchand as we take a cab to the hospital. Poor Aiden, with his big eyes asking me why I was going back to hospital—it broke my heart. We make it in and they are expecting me. I ask quickly for a dish in case I get sick. I am feeling more and more nauseous and my head pounds. I don't even know what to feel emotionally, as I feel so physically sick. I do not want to be back here, that I know for sure.

After being admitted to the ER and having a CT scan, which shows nothing abnormal, I have a lumbar puncture.

I now know after keeping up to date with scientific literature on colloid cysts, that it was okay to have a lumbar puncture, as my colloid cyst no longer existed. If you do have a colloid cyst, especially if you have raised intracranial pressure, you should be very aware of this before having any lumbar punctures as it could lead to brain herniation.[13]

Unfortunately, because my cerebrospinal fluid (CSF) after surgery was so low, they battle to get the needle in for the lumbar puncture. Eventually, they get the CSF sample. I am re-admitted to hospital— back to the neurosurgery intermediary care unit, but not to ICU. It is 10:30 pm.

"Please can you now give me something for the headache?" I get the heart monitors put on my chest again and then the IV Fentanyl, which makes me feel like I am on a cloud wrapped in a warm blanket. The pain goes away and I feel warm and comfy. All is good as I fade off to sleep...

It seems I have chemical or aseptic meningitis,[14] which is basically acute meningitis caused by anything other than the bacteria that typically cause acute bacterial meningitis. Scientific gibberish, I know. As it is not bacterial, I don't get antibiotics. However, I am back on dexamethasone via IV and in hospital for the next two days to ensure I improve. My poor dad, back in Vancouver, is in a flat panic as all he heard was the word meningitis. As soon as the hour is decent, I call him to let him know I am okay and what this type of meningitis is all about. It seems we won't be heading back to Vancouver any time soon.

---

13 Focus on Neuroimaging: Neurology Self-Assessment (Neurology Self-Assessment Series) by Espinosa MD MPH, Patricio S., Smith MD, Charles D. (2009) p 121.

14 http://www.merckmanuals.com/professional/neurologic_disorders/meningitis/overview_of_meningitis.html

Ten

SLEDGEHAMMER

September 10

Email to family and friends

Hi there,

Yes it is me, the real blond one! Just to update you on my condition, I was readmitted to hospital last night after having had a 24-hour migraine. They did a CT scan and lumbar puncture (dug around for gold it seems/feels!). Basically, I may have chemical/aseptic meningitis, which can happen post brain surgery. I was given some lovely medication last night and slept well and it took the edge off the headache and I went to lala land! Saw my neurosurgeon at 5:30 am and then the surgical residents (they work hard) and will be in overnight tonight again as they continue to give me steroids and monitor my condition. Hoping tomorrow will bring a new day! Aiden is definitely more interested in what dad id doing—I am getting very little bandwidth from him.

(Note: when I added this email to the book, I noticed the spelling was bizarre and I could see the effect of the medications in my words!).

On my first night in hospital I am admitted into a double room on the neuro ward with a lady who has just had a stroke. During that night and after hearing her complete confusion, frustration and inability to converse, I get some insight into the devastation of a stroke. I know the acute phase of stroke management is critical. They eventually have to strap her down as she is pulling out all her IV lines and more. The second night, I get put into another double room. From the oxycodone they have given me for pain relief, I have wild delusions that the hospital is actually just a warehouse. I ask the nurse how they will get our blood to the main hospital. I had also started reading *The Hunger Games* on my kindle. Now try that out, *The Hunger Games* with oxycodone. Between thinking Aiden was in *The Hunger Games* and other bizarre thoughts, I drift off to sleep.

By the beginning of day two in hospital, my headaches and nausea are abating. They take the stitches out from my surgery, which is great. But by the end of day two, I feel a headache coming on; slightly different from the one when I was admitted. Oh well, I am sure my head is just complaining about all this attention, I tell myself. After having the hundredth neuro examination, I am discharged, hoping I don't need to step foot in the hospital again.

We finally get back to the hotel, déjà vu, and I am thrilled to be able to give my mom and Aiden a hug. I have not seen them since I was admitted to hospital the second time. There is nothing like the smell of your own child, their cheek against yours. It's pure heaven. The sheer peace of running my own bath and lying in it until my body melts into the bubbles makes me feel heaps better.

But that niggling headache, that I thought was just my brain complaining, is getting worse. Maybe I should have mentioned it to them in hospital, but I am so tired of being tired and mentioning the smallest complaint. I am sure it will be gone by the morning.

September 13

When I wake up the next morning I feel good. It must have just been a headache, nothing more. But as I start to get up and move around, my head starts to pound. I have been upright for a while, having breakfast and then suddenly I feel that I have to lie down. I am nauseous and have the beginnings of a splitting migraine. Within about ten minutes of lying down, the headache eases without any medication. This is bizarre. Until I remember once reading something about lumbar puncture headaches.[15] I read a bit online and everything points to a headache resulting from that series of lumbar punctures before I was admitted for meningitis. Not sure what to do, I call Dr. Q. They advise me to eat food with salt and to drink caffeine, and if it does not improve in a day or two, they may do a blood patch. That does not sound like something I want.

Email to family and friends

Hello all,

Well, am hoping to see the neurosurgeon at 1 pm tomorrow and we are then booked back to Toronto tomorrow night and then on to Vancouver Saturday morning. Hoping this all remains intact as really keen to be home, but at the same time want to ensure we are ready to travel. It has been two weeks since we arrived in Baltimore and how the time has flown. Looking forward to continuing to make a good recovery at home in my bed, with my tea cup in hand :) Mom and Dad will be around for a while longer to help out, which has been amazing given the timing of everything.

Chat soon

---

15 INDICATIONS: Severe, persistent spinal headaches for more than two days after a spine procedure (e.g. epidural steroid injection, myelogram, lumbar puncture) despite conservative treatment. Spinal headaches consist of severe throbbing head pain that starts one day after a spinal procedure. The th obbing occurs with standing and disappears after a few minutes of lying supine. The init al treatment should consist of fluids and est prior to treating with a blood patch. https://www.radiology.wisc.edu/sections/msk/interventional/Blood%20patches%20for%20csf%20leaks/index.php)

So my diet for the next day consists of salted chips and pretzels, lattes with extra shots and some caffeine tablets. So, tonight I have decided to take some of the caffeine tablets and an oxycodone for the headache. I then realize this is the worst combination ever, with the vivid and bizarre hallucinogenic dreams that follow. My body is trying to go to sleep with the oxycodone but is then bumped back awake by the caffeine. It is the 'trip' of a lifetime!

The next day, I take it really easy and lie down most of the day in the hope that this will all just go away. I think by now we are all tired of thinking we are going to leave and then having a medical calamity pop up that delays our return home. Air Canada must love us, given the number of times we have changed our flights. At least the hotel we are staying at knows our story and staff have been so accommodating with our schedule and requests. In fact, the staff all knows Aiden by now. Everyone greets us all by name in the elevator, front desk or coffee shop. Quite funny, really, and they even gave Aiden a Baltimore Orioles baseball team t-shirt as a gift to wear.

Tonight we walked lazily to dinner but within twenty minutes of or-dering, I can barely sit upright—the headache is unbearable. My body knows exactly what it wants to do to correct the situation: lie down. And so I do. We have takeaway dinner in the hotel room, me lying down and eating.

By the following day we are seeing no dramatic improvement. I just want to go home, and I am not the only one. The neurosurgical team has suggested coming in for a blood patch. If that relieves the headaches, I will then be cleared to fly home the next day. Medicine is amazing. To be honest I feel a bit nervous about going back to the hospital for the third time since we arrived here, but know I will be in good hands.

Text message to my husband

Dear Marchand,

You are my star and I always can count on you. You amaze me with your patience, love and never-ending compassion. Thank you for everything my love.

I love u more than anything in this world.

Tiny

Marchand and I take a cab again to the hospital. We now know the route by heart and go straight to the ambulatory surgical unit. All I can do is sprawl myself horizontally across the chair to get my head level to the ground. I feel like one of those construction tools with the water balance bubble that needs to be at a certain angle.

They call us through to the OR. I am given a bed in the intake section—this looks so familiar from the day I had my brain surgery. The anesthesiologist who looked after me for my surgery is there and is obviously surprised to see me again.

In order to figure out if a blood patch will work for me, the anesthesiologist on call gives me a huge bear hug and squeezes me as tight as possible around my stomach area. He asks me to let him know when the headache stops.

Lo and behold, a few moments later, I felt a relief from the headache. "Now," I say.

As soon as he let go, the throbbing, searing headache came back. I lay back against the pillow, desperate to be horizontal.

"Yes, this definitely looks like a CSF leak, I think a blood patch[16] is needed here. Let me go talk to Dr. Q as I am currently assisting him in a surgery".

And so, after more IV lines, fentanyl for the pain and procedure, and blood taken (about 45 ml from my veins) and put into the catheter

16 An epidural blood patch is a surgical procedure that provides immediate relief to the headache caused by leaking spinal fluid. pproximately 15-20 mls of blood is taken from a vein in the patient's arm and subsequently injected into the epidural space in the spine at the site of the spinal fluid l ak. (http://www.epidural.net/blood-patch.htm)

around my spine, all is done. The anesthesiologist says there was definitely a leak, as he put in a lot of blood into the spine area before it gave resistance. I lie in the warm fentanyl blanket fog for about thirty minutes, vaguely aware of my husband having a conversation with the anesthesiologist about yachts and mining.

After thirty minutes, it is time to see if this works. They slowly put my bed upright to see if the headache returns.

Please... I beg... let this work.

Nothing. No headache, only a throbbing in my back from all the prodding and the patch. We are done and if I have no headache tomorrow morning when I wake, we can get on that plane and fly home. *Hasta la vista*, baby! That sounds like the best thing ever.

Dr. Q has finished his surgery and comes by again to say hi. What a man he is. Compassionate, and carrying printouts of all my medical records for me to take home. After everything we have been through, he just makes it all so much easier.

We say goodbye, hopefully for the last time, to Johns Hopkins Bayview Medical Center and head back to the hotel. Although I am hoping not to have to come here again, I am so very grateful this is where we did come as we received the best care possible.

September 14

Email to family and friends

Had blood patch so only flying tomorrow but great care again at hospital! Out for dinner... Then early bed:)

Lots of love

Claire

Sledgehammer

Facebook post

Home approved tomorrow afternoon as had blood patch on spine for post lumbar puncture headache! Dinner in tum, off to bed and ready for home! Lots of love to u all.

My body is so tired of needles and the smell of antiseptic and anesthetic. My arms are painful and riddled with bruises; my back is now sore from the blood patch. My mind knows I have made it through, this will come right. Now I just want to cyber space it home, one quick trip, not two planes and an overnight stay.

September 15

We are now half way home. We are in Toronto at the airport hotel having dinner, and I am ravenous. It's a good sign, I think. *(Little will I know that this was only the beginning of my monstrous dexametha-sone-fuelled appetite!)* Tomorrow is the flight home.

I cannot wait to get home. To see my dad, my house, make my own cuppa tea and I know it is time for Aiden to be back with his buddies, to be in school and for Marchand to be back at work. Life goes on and for us that is a reality we are ready for.

I wake up in the middle of the night and my head feels like it in space, it feels like it is floating and aching. Healing is probably the right word for it. But in order to sleep better, I get a t-shirt and wrap it around my head. It feels better. Of course Marchand gets a good laugh out of this when he wakes up. I will definitely have to look for a toque/beanie to wear to bed when I get home. Stylish? Not! Comfy and essential, yes! I find, just like when I am feeling sick, there is nothing like a warm duvet to wrap around your body to make you feel better. I suppose my head deserves the same.

As we fly over beautiful Canada and the majestic scenery below, we start to head towards Vancouver. I stand up in the galley-way and look out the window at the snow-capped mountains and water as far as the eye can see. Land of water and wilderness. I feel an overwhelming emotion pass through my body; the tears just start to come. I cannot stop them. All the fear, anger, and happiness of the past three weeks comes tumbling out as I realize that I am almost home, almost done with this journey.

My mom comes to find me and puts her arms around me. She tells me "It's okay to cry. You have been through so much, and I am so proud of you."

As we descend into Vancouver, Aiden tries to comfort me from the tears by handing me the stuffed husky dog we got him in Toronto. At the arrivals area there is something incredibly special about being wheeled through to see my dad, whom I have not seen in almost three weeks. He has tears in his eyes. I am so happy to see him and I can see how tremendously relieved he is to see us all. This whole journey has been a hard one for all of us in the US, but at the same time incredibly hard for him being alone in Vancouver, awaiting news.

It is so good to have everyone back together; the healing can now really begin for us all.

Eleven

HOMEWARD BOUND

September 16

Facebook post

Landed Vancouver! Loving the sun out the window ☺

People have been so kind. We arrive home to lots of flowers and even a few hats and beanies for me. I realize now that people thought I would have a lot of hair shaved off and thinking back, so would I have thought that! But you can hardly tell I had brain surgery as the incision line is behind my hairline and by combing my fringe (bangs) forward, you can hardly even see it. However, we are heading into fall and the beanies are most welcome as my skull can now feel every drop in temperature.

My dear friend Melissa has already been hard at work and baked lasagna awaits our arrival at home. I always knew she was a gem, but will come to realize over the coming months how kind and generous she really is. Best friends are integral to one's recovery and I am lucky to be able to count a few of these on my hand.

September 17

It takes me a while to get back into the routine of being at home. It feels so quiet after the hustle and bustle of the hospital and hotel. I love my cuppa tea and for me the small act of making a pot of tea feels like heaven, almost a meditation. Aiden is now back to school; he missed two weeks while we were in Baltimore. The poor little chap woke us up last night in tears, as he was scared and nervous about going back to school. I think also, an accumulation of uncertainty, fear and the unknown was included in the tears that streamed down his face.

Our first day home and I have a follow-up appointment with my new neurosurgeon at the large hospital downtown. My GP organized the appointment while we were away. He was the neurosurgeon I saw for a second opinion two years ago, who said I must definitely continue with yearly MRIs. He has an outstanding reputation. I will continue to be monitored now as his patient with yearly follow up MRI's for the time being. His one statement to me took me by surprise; he said to be prepared for up to a one-year recovery from this surgery. One year! That is forever. I have things to do, work to get back to—not sure I can wait a year to feel better. But I suppose it takes time for the brain to heal.

I love still having my mom and dad around—not that I am spending much time with them. My bed and I are intertwined for about twenty hours out of the twenty-four-hour day. Fatigue floods every fiber and cell of my being. I sleep and then wake up, walk slowly downstairs, see my folks, and maybe sit outside with my cup of tea, as the weather is still lovely. And then within an hour or two my body starts to feel heavy and it is back to bed. I am now three weeks post op. This routine will continue for at least the next two weeks. I feel like my body has lead weights on my feet and I need an arm to hold onto if we are out and about—I do not yet feel steady enough to walk by myself.

Each evening, we stroll slowly down the road to the beach and back, husband's commands in order to keep my body moving—good idea. I can now measure my change in stamina by how I feel once I get to the end of the road. It is slowly getting better. To feel this as an adult is refreshing yet frustrating at the same time. It's strange to start all over again and not be able to walk more than twenty meters down the road without having to turn around to come home.

Yet the next day, I can maybe do a twenty-two-meter shuffle. My progress and recovery are being played out before my very eyes on the road before me in feet. Literally. How very important it is to keep moving, even in small steps. It helps with other things. It helps me keep my body more mobile and prevents other issues cropping up. It gives me fresh air to breathe, and time to be grateful for the wonderful view at the end of the road, and for the precious time with my parents who help me to walk each day.

I am thrilled that Aiden is back at school. It is so important that he is back into his routine and seeing his buddies. He is happy and it brings him a sense of structure and security.

Dad is going to go back home next week. He was on his own here in Vancouver for almost three weeks while we were in Baltimore; his back is really painful and he needs to have further investigations. Mom will stay on for another week or two, until she and I feel I can manage on my own. I find that during the day it is reassuring to have my parents in the house. I am able to get around by myself, but I am so tired. They also fetch Aiden from school and sort him out in the afternoon until Marchand gets home, as I am just not able to muster up that much energy. Between Mom and Dad doing the grocery shopping and Marchand being MasterChef, we have food on the table. Mom helps out with keeping the never-ending laundry cycle going, so we have clean clothes. Dad continues to walk Bolt each day so the dog is happy. Therefore, the house seems to be running smoothly at this point in time.

I am not 100 percent sure how to feel about a comment made to me today: "I am sure you feel blessed and grateful that it was not cancer, it makes it so much easier." I couldn't agree more. I have had that thought many times myself as the reality of the past weeks has sunk in. However, now being on the receiving end of such a comment, it feels strange, and even though well-intended and true, it hurt.

But as time would pass and wounds would heal, I would realize that my journey through brain surgery was only half of what many patients with brain cancer go through and this would make my determination to do something to contribute towards this area even more important. That would spur on my fundraising and eventually start this book. Later on in my recovery, I would understand that comments like this come up because people often don't realize that non-malignant tumors can still be life-threatening. They don't say it to be mean, but with good intentions.

I have not really had many visitors at home as I am hardly awake for long enough to be sociable! One of our dearest friends, Nicole, and her son pop over for a brief visit. We have known each other since South Africa and our husbands work together. Old friends who stand the test of time, as they say. Their family is basically like our family here in Vancouver, since our relatives are all in South Africa, and our boys are true mates. It is so lovely to see them and catch up, although I feel as if I'm in a fog and up in a cloud. After ten minutes, my brain starts to shut down. Socializing time is up! This is obviously something I will have to retrain myself to do. After my strenuous twenty-minute coffee with a friend, I need to have a nap straight away. Yipes!

September 19

My short-term memory seems to be affected both by the heavy fatigue and from the surgery and the fog of medications. I keep a notepad and pen next to my bed to write down anything I need to remember as well as keep lists in my iPhone. Nothing seems to stick in my brain. It is like I need post-it notes stuck all over the house to remember things I need to do even just when I walk from one room to another to do something! Well, I suppose my brain has had a massive assault on it, just give it time to heal and calm down.

Note in my iPhone to myself

I have been blessed by love, by family, by friends, by time and by space. Not so much by health today but I still count each and every blessing before closing my eyes at night as I know how lucky I am to be able to have them.

Well now, let's change the topic and talk about my appetite. It's better than it's ever been in my life. I am constantly hungry and my face in the mirror is getting noticeably round. Hmm.

I read up more about the steroid I am on, dexamethasone, as I am sure I remember seeing something about this in the medication leaflet I got when I left hospital. Some of the listed side effects are increased appetite and a round or full face. I seem to definitely be suffering from these. But I am due to finish my course of dexamethasone this week, so I am sure it will not take long for my face to stop looking like a moon and for my voracious appetite to calm down. I am also taking Keppra to prevent seizures (seems to be standard procedure post brain surgery), an antiemetic (to prevent nausea) and standard Tylenol for any pain or headaches. The oxycodone is only for when I need to pull out the big guns to target a really bad headache or pain that is not being resolved with the Tylenol. Not there yet! I remember the hallucinations that I had with that in hospital so I am trying to stay away from it unless necessary.

September 21

Without being melodramatic, thanks to this man for helping me out this time three weeks ago and bringing me home safe and sound! A very interesting and inspiring story of an illegal immigrant who has become one of the leading neurosurgeons in his field—his ability to care for patients as a person and a doctor is amazing: http://doctorqmd.com/assets/files/1/files/pdfs/quinones_baltimore_nov2011-.pdf

I have also purchased Dr. Q's book, *Becoming Dr. Q: My Journey From Migrant Farm Worker to Brain Surgeon*. I am so interested to find out more about his journey after reading this article I found on his website about him.

I am finally able to pop the last dexamethasone tablet down the gullet—yippee! Something quite gratifying about getting off all these medications; it feels like a step in the right direction. Unfortunately, I wake up the next morning with a splitting headache, a band across my head. I am nauseous with the pain. What?

Now I bring in the big guns, it's oxycodone to the rescue. Nothing seems to work, though, and by the next day we call Johns Hopkins to ask them what to do. I cannot even get out of bed, the headache is so bad.

Once again the team at Johns Hopkins call me back within ten minutes of me leaving a message and they say that I should head to the local ER to get a CT scan. I see my poor husband sink to the floor and swear at it all. I feel the same. I can see that this is the last thing Marchand needs; we are just getting things back together and now. Marchand wonders if this headache is linked to me finishing my dexamethasone medication the other day.

Just as we consider the way ahead, my cell phone goes off. It is Johns Hopkins again. They have called Dr. Q (this is a Sunday) and he thinks it could be a dexamethasone-withdrawal issue. They advise that rather than heading to the ER in my infection-prone post-surgical state, I should head to the local GP and get more dexamethasone. I am to take it immediately and, if no relief overnight, then head straight to the ER.

We head off to the local clinic to see a GP and as I fulfill my new script for dexamethasone, the pharmacist asks me if I have ever taken this medication before. She called it a 'dirty drug' due to the range of side effects that some people can get from this medication. I could not agree more; the side effects are not great but I know it is essential. It seems my body needs more time to adjust to weaning off this 'dirty drug.'

We get home and I gulp down the dexamethasone and pray it will sort out my headache. Sleep and dexamethasone and an oxy—that should do the trick.

By the next day, I am feeling much better. So in a conference call with Dr. Q, my GP and I chat and figure out the best way forward. Dr. Q recommends a very slow wean off dexamethasone; some people struggle to get off it more than others. At the slower rate it will take me another two months to get off the medication but if that is what it takes, then that is what it will take. I am not going to screw around with this.

It does mean that the "Feed me Seymour" monster in my tummy is going to be around for a while longer. The craving for carbohydrates and food all through the day is insane. Over the course of my dexamethasone feast (three months in total), I will put on over five kilograms and have a face like a moon. Dexamethasone also seems to deposit fat right in your abdominal area and the back of the neck area. I can attest to that and, although I might be slight of frame and build, my body feels so different. I know that time will pass, and I will eventually be able to exercise more and it will sort itself out, I hope. The dexamethasone also gives me lots of joint pain, especially in my knees and hips and lower back. The combination of having been in surgery and immobile for so long, with taking a drug like dexamethasone, means it is just one of those things that will happen. So, I try to keep mobile with gentle walks, use heat packs for the pain and know that time will pass.

I have realized that I will need to get some after-school help for Aiden for when my mom has returned home: someone to fetch him from school, bring him home and look after him until Marchand is home from work. I am not yet driving and also still napping in the afternoon, and have not yet got enough energy under my belt to cope with Aiden by myself in the afternoons. Who would have thought?

I search online nanny agencies to no avail. Before my dad leaves, he suggests I look at agencies that cater to the senior care category—they tend to offer care options on a short-term basis when people need a few hours here and there. I contact as many agencies as I can and get a huge response. Thank goodness, I eventually find what I am looking for. This is good to know for future use.

It is interesting how my needs have changed, and waxed and waned throughout my journey with my colloid cyst. For example, in the beginning when I was asking loads of questions and trying to understand everything, I visited the colloid cyst Facebook group every single day. As I felt more comfortable with the condition, I then found the depth of information regarding post-op outcomes and questions to be over-whelming for me. So I took a little break from reading the posts. Then I started dropping back in again every so often to see what was going on and started reconnecting with people. When I started to get sick in August, and now after surgery, this group has been a lifeline for me—a place where people, both pre and post op, give moral support and positive enforcement as well as personal answers to questions on a daily basis. Thanks, Facebook group!

Support groups are such an integral part of a recovery process. If you can find a support group, whether online or in your community, it is worthwhile looking into. Being able to hear other people's stories and experiences, as well as sharing your own, is extremely helpful. Try to connect with your national Brain Tumor Foundation or Network if one exists to see what support tools they can offer you as well. No matter how much our loved ones and friends love us and empathize with us, speaking to a fellow survivor can be very enlightening, therapeutic and ease the burden.

What do my days look like one month post surgery?

I am taking everything really slowly. I get up very slowly in the morning; have a big nap (two hours before lunch and then another nap in the afternoon. Bedtime calls early for me, around 8 pm. So sleeping is still a major contributor to my daily activities. During the day, I catch up on a few emails but don't spend much time on the computer; I find it quite tiring. I lie down and read or just zone out. I am not yet driving, so my mom drives me around for my doctor's appointments if needed. She also helps out with fetching Aiden from school. Once she goes home, that role will be taken over by the caregiver for the next month or two, depending on how my recovery goes. Help around the house with cooking, laundry, cleaning and everything else has been tremendous otherwise everything would have come to a grinding halt.

I have now finished all my medications except for the dexamethasone. It is still early days, too early to really say how I feel. But I am here and grateful for that. I'm moving forward, with small steps. That is the main thing.

Twelve

FINDING THE 'NEW NORMAL'

October 22

People often ask me: "Were you scared before your surgery?" To be honest, I was not. However, I think this was entirely due to the fact that I was feeling so out of it. My body was slowly fading, my memory was worsening and I was exhausted. The long plane trip and journey to Johns Hopkins was about all that I could handle. There was one moment when I did start to feel anxious, when things seemed real. This was right before they put me under the general anesthetic. Over the past seven years, I have had over four general anesthetics and each time, I have felt more and more nervous just before they put me to sleep. So, now I ask someone to hold my hand when it is that time. Somehow, that physical link to the world around me helps takes away my fear.

The month of October has been an interesting one for me. During the first week, Mom left to go back home. We decided that I was ready enough to be on my own during the day and I found a caregiver to

97

fetch Aiden from school and look after him for a few hours after school while I was napping. The support structures were all in place.

Later in October, I also took to the wheel of my car again. I was no longer on any medications that could impact my driving and had been cleared over four weeks ago to drive. How liberating! I feel like a teenager again, doing my learners, that excitement and anticipation of taking the first drive alone. I had not driven in over two months.

This weekend we all hopped in the car and took a drive up to the shops, only two kilometers up the hill.

As I pulled into the parking space at the shops and stopped the car, I pulled the keys out the ignition and giggled like a child, "I did it, yippee, Yay!"

"Well done, Mom!" said Aiden. Another small celebration for a big step for me.

And so the small steps continue. I start driving here and there and then driving Aiden to school again in the mornings. It makes me feel much more competent and part of the human race again.

Apart from seeing my GP on a more regular basis to monitor my dexamethasone-tapering regime and general health post surgery, the other health care professionals that I have sought out to assist me in my recovery at this stage are my naturopath, massage therapist and chiropractor.

My naturopath has always helped me out with my multivitamin and mineral regime and we are now adding a few things to help my body out in its time of healing. As I have an arthritic hip, I see a massage therapist on a monthly basis anyway. Since my surgery, I have found my body is protesting loudly. My back and neck and body ache. I think my general immobility adds to the issue, so my massage therapist and chiropractor are both an integral part of keeping me moving. A holistic approach, I think, is an important part to my body's overall recovery. However, before seeing either of them I got an all-clear from my neurosurgeon.

It is now two months post-surgery and even now, napping and being vigilant about mapping out my days and energy expenditure are a vital part in how I fare by the end of the day. To Aiden's delight I am able to volunteer for the Halloween party at school and dress up. But I have to plan it out. I have to nap beforehand and then still come home and hand him over to the caregiver and go straight to bed for a two-hour nap. *C'est la vie.* Instead of planning our lives around a toddler's naps and schedule these days, it is around my naps and schedule – remember those days? Funny how life happens, right? My body consumes hours of sleep like there is no tomorrow.

The fatigue that I feel after this surgery is like no other fatigue that I have ever experienced. I have had chronic anemia, been pregnant, sleep deprived and much more. But this type of fatigue grips every fiber of my body. It takes hold of my brain at the same time and I can literally feel it turn the switch off inside my head. And at that moment, the power grid goes off.

November 14

The tears still come, sometimes prompted by the smallest thing. I feel like it is a reminder of what has happened and how lucky I am to still be here to experience this. The extreme fatigue and slight dizziness is also frustrating. I feel as if someone has pressed the pause button in my life.

I now know that my body can only handle so much. Whenever I 'overdo' it, I pay the consequences of extreme exhaustion for days afterwards. The sad thing is that the overdoing it is usually something small that would not normally have even been an issue. I keep reminding myself that the biggest thing about brain surgery is the fatigue, and that with time my normal energy levels should return. So for now, I just need to learn to accept living at a slower pace, putting less pressure on myself than I used to and knowing that one day, things will be back to normal, or a new form of 'normal' for me. It is only just over two months post-surgery; I am still an infant in this whole process.

Now that my parents are back in South Africa and it is just me at home during the day, I have decided it is time to take the plunge. It is time to get back to try and walk the seawall. This is my favorite walk along the seaside near our house. Each time I have walked it the past, it has been a different experience. I have walked it in the radiant sunshine, the gentle and not-so-gentle rain, in flurries of snow and dense fog so thick that all I can see is five meters in front of me. I have walked it with friends and family and by myself. But each time, I feel like I have had added fifteen minutes to my life. The fresh air, the lovely scenery and the fluid lines between the modern bustling world and nature are seamless.

So, today is the day that I put my trainers back on my feet and try the seawall again. Since being home and doing my five-minute walks down the road at the end of each day, my body craves the steady and regular motion of one step forward. Walking on a regular basis has helped make me feel stronger in a very measured way.

Note to self: the seawall is a five-kilometer walk and today my aim is to walk for ten minutes only and then turn around. That is all! I am starting with small steps as I have already learned the consequences of overdoing the most simple of tasks. The air is as fresh as I remember, the views as lovely and this time my heart is overjoyed. I feel as if I have won the lottery. I am here, I am in the moment and I am walking. By myself. On the seawall. After brain surgery. This is it!

After ten minutes I turn around, already starting to feel tired but knowing I am on the right track. I finish my walk and phone my mom back in South Africa:

"Mom, I just walked for twenty minutes on the seawall!" I feel tears on my face. This time, they are tears of joy. As adults, we don't often feel that wonder of achieving something so big with something so small. The wonder that young children feel on a daily basis that makes their lives so full of smiles is really special. I probably only walked one kilometer today, but the elation and triumph I felt was more than when I surpassed the eighteen-kilometer mark on my half-marathon training.

This would be a true lesson from this journey: I would come to appreciate taking great joy from the smallest accomplishments in my life. I can only hope I can take this lesson forward with me.

While I may be feeling grateful about so many aspects in my life at present, the one emotion that has taken me by surprise is anger. I am not an angry person by nature. Yet at the moment, I have a lot of anger inside me: anger that I was misdiagnosed in my referral hospital.

This feeling is so intense some days as I struggle to accept that this could happen to another parent of a young child. If a patient did not have the money to get the surgery done elsewhere, what would happen to them? As I lie down and close my eyes to nap and go to sleep, these feelings flood my thoughts and I struggle to push them aside.

Marchand and I have refused to sit idle and potentially let this happen to someone else. So we have spoken to a dear friend of ours who is a lawyer and his advice was to determine our key objective. Are we trying to recover the finances spent in this surgery, or ensure that the doctors acknowledged that the outcome was not medically correct and should have been handled differently?

We realize that our key objective is to ensure that this type of thing does not happen to someone else. Our secondary objective is to try and retrieve some of the funds spent on the out of country surgery. So, after much discussion, we decided to file complaints against the doctors concerned with the College of Physicians and Surgeons of

British Columbia. The case file will take me quite a while to complete. Firstly, as I am still recovering from surgery and it is tiring and will take my brain a while to figure out all the requirements. Secondly, as there are so many details that I want to ensure are taken into account when the Board assesses this case.

I know that after filing my complaint, I will feel more at ease. I know if I don't pursue this course of action, it will always stay in the back of my mind as a "what if." It is best for me to deal with things head on and then lay them to rest so that we can all move on.

I have also realized just how much my folks and Marchand have done for me over the past months, hence I put together a few words as well as a photo collage for each of them to let them know that their thoughts and actions have not gone unnoticed while all the focus and attention has been on me.

This is a tribute to my Mom and Dad
For all their kindness and patience
For their support without being asked
Their love and guidance
Boardwalk strolls in Baltimore
Cups of Hong Kong tea
Time with Aiden outside in our garden or at Parc Verdun
Yam fries and a beautiful view
All these are blessings I will never take for granted.

This is a tribute to my husband.
For all his love for Aiden and me, through anything
For his patience
His kind heart, which seems to know no boundaries
His ability to be strong no matter what comes our way...
This amazes me

His sense of humor, bringing a smile to my face
The thoughtful acts of everyday kindness making it so worthwhile
Watching him as a father, love his son
Makes me feel whole
Knowing all these things about him
Makes me feel special and lucky
I count my blessings each and every night before I close my eyes...
He is the first.

What do my days look like three months post surgery?

Not that much has changed, to be honest. My body still craves sleep like I would not have thought possible and I still need to nap after lunch each day for 1-2 hours. However, I don't need to nap in the mornings anymore. I am awake when Aiden gets back from school but need a top-up shorter nap around 3 pm to get through the rest of the afternoon. My body itself is still aching in very strange places, e.g. neck and back, but I am trying to keep as mobile as I can as I think the immobility is part of the issue. My appetite is really good, due to the dexamethasone, so no issues there. No pain medications needed. My emotions are a bit fragmented, possibly due to the fatigue, and the frustration that comes with it.

This is a topic that I was not sure where to place in my book but I know it comes up in many discussions in our group and I am experiencing it right now. I would say that I am generally a pretty confident person in life. Yes, I get scared by some things, nervous before presentations and sometimes doubt myself. I think that is normal.

I have, however, noticed that since my surgery, I am not as confident as I was before. I am not sure if this stems from the fact that my life has been turned upside down and now has to be so much more regimented to allow me to keep control and keep my stamina and energy levels up. I know that I am way more in tune with my body than I have ever been in my life, but at the same time, I am more cautious than I ever used to be. For example, I ask myself, "what will the effect of this activity have on the rest of today and tomorrow and the week?"

It might also be that my short-term memory is not what it used to be; I forget faces and words or my train of thought more regularly than I used to. My stamina is lower, so I don't feel as confident to carry out the task or stay the extra hour at a play date. The combination of all these things means that my level of confidence in myself is diminished. I feel more of a wallflower than I used to, but at the same time I feel more conspicuous. I look normal to everyone from the outside but on the inside, the wires seem to be crossed. I have moments when I feel shy, like I used to at school. For goodness sake, I am an adult now, no need to go back to those insecurities—but they come flooding back.

I saw a lovely saying today that I really took to heart: "What other people think of me is none of my business." I don't know whether this lack of confidence will fade with time. I do hope so, as this is not who I truly am, not who I am used to being. It is hard, as not everyone around me will really understand how this feels. Having your brain operated on does more than give you an ache in your head.

This would all start to make sense to me later in my recovery, when I would consult a clinical psychologist who opened the door and shed some light on the dark recesses of my brain and its secrets.

December 5

The countdown is now on for Christmas. Once Halloween is over, the next day the shops seem to be festooned with red, green and Rudolph. I do love this time of year, though, especially in the Northern Hemisphere. There is something so special about experiencing Christmas in the cold. It feels right.

Finding the 'New Normal'

We are staying in Vancouver for December, given our summer extravagance of two out-of-country trips—one unintended, for sure! We have lunches and festive celebrations planned with close friends who are our family; at this time of year a lot of us celebrate without family close by.

Slowly, slowly, my energy is returning. I still nap each day after lunch and take it slow, but I can feel I am heading in the right direction. It has now been just over three and a half months since my surgery. I can't believe it; it feels like it was only two months ago. Time is not my enemy, my mind is. Some days my body feels like it is swimming through mud and other days, through thick water. It just depends. One weird thing is that I feel like my body thermostat is confused. I sweat like a beast. I must chat to my GP about it when I next see her; I'm not sure it means anything, but boy, is it irritating and embarrassing. Hormonal, maybe?

Since I work for myself, we have decided to take it very much day by day to see when the right time is to return to work. I feel blessed that I am not on a rigid time line. Right now I know my body and mind are definitely not ready to work. Not sure napping and working fit together at this point. I love working and know I will just push myself hard, so the time needs to be right.

Thirteen

ONE STEP BACK

December 23

The darkness is thick. My eyes open; I am not sure why I have woken up. I turn to look at my phone and the unwelcome yet familiar feeling of the room spinning engulfs me.

My fear speaks first: please, no. I thought this was all gone.

I gently get out of bed and as I do, I feel as though I have stepped off a merry-go-round. The vague outline of the bed looms before me, moving in circles and from side to side. I stumble to the washroom just as I am about to be sick. I hover around the toilet, waiting. Nothing. I glance up at the ceiling, which is now moving in a sickening dance above me. Please, no.

Maybe this is a nightmare and I will wake up soon. I damn well hope so, as I have just started, literally this Sunday, to feel the life come back into my body and my personality start to shine a little. It is almost four months since my surgery. I count the minutes and then try to stand up from the bathroom floor, not so easy when you feel you are in a boat in the middle of a storm. I head downstairs, take a Serc and head back upstairs to the safety of my bed to try and sleep this out. It is the twenty-third of December. Is this my early Christmas present?

December 25

I have spent a lot of time lying down and sleeping the past two days. This vertigo attack has sapped the life of out me once again. Maybe it is because my body is still in recovery mode. I am so lucky that Marchand has taken Christmas and New Year off work so he is around to help out while I will my body back to life. We spend Christmas Day with our Vancouver 'family' who are our dear friends and have a lovely day eating, chatting and enjoying each other's company. Of course, I take two naps upstairs during the course of the day. I am feeling worse and worse since my vertigo attack. My fatigue is heavier, my limbs are numb, I am dizzy.

December 28

My GP orders blood tests to see if anything shows up. It shows elevated TSH (thyroid stimulating hormone, elevated cortisol and low ferritin). So this may explain why I feel like I am swimming in mud. I have a mild anemia and hypothyroidism at present and my cortisol is high—my body is still in stress response mode. Once again, she urges me to visit the ER if I do not see a marked improvement in my symptoms.

December 31

New Years Eve for me has lost the enticement of staying up till the wee hours of the morning and sipping away on a few too many glasses of wine—especially this year, since bedtime is 7:30 pm. As for wine, I cannot drink more than a tot without feeling drunk. We have tried! So it is early bed for us all, and I hope I wake up tomorrow feeling like a new woman. Please give me a makeover—that is my New Year's wish!

January 1

Hmm, not sure my New Year's wish got fulfilled. I feel even worse today and since Marchand has to actually go back to work soon, we head off to the ER for a checkup. It is 7 am on New Year's Day. We are bound to see some interesting sights in the ER this morning that is for sure! We head downtown to the hospital where my neurosurgeon is based. Amazingly, the ER is quiet. Aiden and Marchand head back into the city to go and do 'boy stuff' while I sit it out and wait to see a doctor.

I see a doctor who does bloods and then a CT scan as well. All looks good, no hydrocephalus. I am relieved. But at the same time, why am I feeling so terrible? No explanation, really. We head home and as we are eating our lunch, I get a call from the doctor at the hospital. She apologizes profusely for asking me to come back in, but a neuro-radiologist has seen something on the CT scan that may explain my vertigo and other symptoms. They would like me to come back in for a CT angiogram[17] (CT angiography uses a CT scanner to produce detailed images of both blood vessels and tissues in various parts of the body e.g. brain). So we head back.

By now, the ER is bursting at the seams. It is 1 pm. I wait patiently and get my CT angiogram done. They warn me that when they inject the dye, I will feel as if I am wetting my pants but not to worry, it is just a feeling—so glad they told me that as it was true—bizarre! I also see the neurologist-on-call with his resident. I did not realize at the time that they were actually the stroke team.

After my neurological exam, which I can do backwards by now, they say that the CT angiogram shows there could have been a stroke in

---

17 CT angiogram: http://www.radiologyinfo.org/en/info.cfm?pg=angioct

the pons area of the brain. But it could also be an artefact, meaning the reflection of the skull. So they have me booked for an MRI at seven tomorrow morning and are admitting me to hospital overnight. No jokes. It is the first of January, and I may have had a stroke. Seriously?

I don't want to alarm Marchand so I just tell him that the quickest way to get an MRI is to book me into hospital overnight. I wait for three hours in the ER waiting room to get a bed with a load of people who by now are spilling out the front doors of the hospital. Anyone who needs to get back to work on the second of January but cannot see his or her local GP is here now. Eventually I get admitted and am taken up to the orthopedic ward, as that is all they have.

Oh well. I must say that I have the most amazing view from the room; I am on the ninth floor and can see the ski hill lights on Grouse Mountain and Cypress twinkling back at me.

It is about 11 pm by the time I get settled into my bed. I stare blankly out the window. I know this is not incredibly serious, otherwise I would not be in the orthopedic ward. However, if I have had a stroke, this is bad news considering I am also recovering from brain surgery. I doze away the night staring out the window at the twinkling lights on the ski hills and the lights in the city. I'm trying to make sense of this all. I then decide that I can't, not until I have the MRI results. There is no sense in worrying about something over which I have no control and no additional information. I decide to try and sleep.

January 2

It is early morning and the mist is just rising over the water of Vancouver. It is breathtaking. I snap away a few pictures on my phone, to remember my start to 2013. The beauty before me makes me feel more positive.

At 6 am they come through to get me to MRI. I have not really slept all night. My mind has not been still. I am trying hard not to get over-anxious about the 'maybe' stroke but cannot believe this would happen now during my recovery, and on New Year's Day, of all days.

The familiar clonking sound of the MRI almost puts me to sleep. Afterwards I am happy to get a breakfast tray, as my food intake over the past twenty-four hours has been sporadic. About two hours after my MRI, my neurologist comes in to say he has just been sitting with the neuro-radiologist going over my MRI. It all looks good. There is definitely no stroke, no hydrocephalus and my brain looks good. They have been over it with a fine tooth comb to ensure they have not overlooked anything.

Thank goodness. I call Marchand and tell him: it's time to go home now, and I want to go home. I call my folks and explain what has been going on in the last twenty-four hours, reassuring them that all is okay. I know it is not easy for them being so far away and unable to do anything.

I spend the next few days sleeping as much as I can and willing my body to switch back into first gear. I know that Marchand needs to go back to the office. He has been amazing at helping out and being at home to help with Aiden.

So the verdict of my hospital visit is that I had a vertigo attack and given my current recovery from brain surgery, my body is simply unable to recover like it used to. It is sapped of all energy. I also have a hormonal quandary going on, as well as the anemia, which is contributing to the immense fatigue. Hopefully some supplementation will help sort that out. Keep on moving forward, two steps!

January 15

Christmas has come and gone, Aiden is back to school, and I continue the climb back up the mountain of recovery after brain surgery. The path sometimes eludes me, sometimes makes me stumble and fall, but at the same time I am proud of my progress.

The good news is that I am finally off my dexamethasone. It has taken four months for my body to agree that it is time to ditch it. Great celebrations all round!

Now that the new year is here and I have recovered from my dizzy spin into it, I have to start studying for my Canadian citizenship exam. I had to postpone my last scheduled date as it was only two months after my surgery and I was not in the right frame of mind to study for it, let alone write an exam. So, now I need to dust off the brain and get going. It will be a good challenge for me and I need to start getting my brain working if I want to return to work.

I am also waiting to see when I will get to see an endocrinologist, due to my elevated cortisol and altered thyroid levels. Given my recent vertigo attack, I am also heading back to see my ENT for a checkup. He reckons I have labyrinthitis (an inflammation of the inner ear which can cause vertigo) and says there's no need to worry, just to keep as active as possible. He says he could send me for balance tests, although given all the testing I have had recently, this might be excessive. I decide I would actually like to go for the balance tests. I no longer like to function in grey areas; knowing things in black and white is much more my comfort zone. Given this is now my third vertigo attack I would like a little further investigation, especially since the 'original suspect' inside my brain is no longer in residence. The waiting list for these balance tests is four months but, because of my surgery, I get rapid placement for two months time! Oh well. Watch and wait, I suppose.

I am now into my fifth month post surgery. I read about other people's recoveries in our group and some are on the same track as I am: still slowly getting their lives back together. Others are back at work with everything 'back to normal'. I find my slow recovery frustrating, but know that I have to listen to my body. After my recent stint in hospital, I know there is no chance my body and brain are ready for a return to work. I am still heavily dependent on my lunchtime nap.

I have made sure to work daily exercise, in some small form, into my regime. Getting my body moving is really important to me so I walk my seawall walk as often as I can. I have also started back at my gym— slowly, but not 100 percent sure if this is a good or bad idea. I will just have to see how my body handles it.

I think recovering from either brain surgery or a brain injury is not something that can be easily quantified. You cannot put a cast on it and estimate that after six weeks, it will be healed and you can then start all activities again. People vary dramatically in the time needed to recover. Individual experiences can also be very different.

But then again, as individuals we are all so different, aren't we? And that is all because of our brains! So, it makes sense that when you are talking about a surgery or injury to the brain, that recovery would be different for each person. Doctors can give a broad framework of what to expect, but it is hard to paint a picture of the quality of life after such an event. I have wondered over and over again if the fact that I had hydrocephalus has played a role in my recovery and will make it take longer than others. Who knows?

The other unique circumstance about recovering from brain surgery or brain injury is that from the outside, you tend to look fine. In fact, you may even look good. You may look just the same as you looked before the surgery. I did. I did not have all my hair shaved off, which most people expected. So, as time passes, and you perhaps are not walking slowly anymore and looking a bit frail, people forget that you had brain surgery. However, behind the scenes, there are a myriad of things going on. That has been really hard for me to deal with sometimes: looking good on the outside, when everything on the inside feels lousy. It is not in my nature to want to be portrayed as the victim.

However, it is hard at the same time to put on a brave face all the time when you look fine but feel exhausted and frail. 'Wearing the mask' as a friend put it, is tiring in itself.

I now understand the risks that come with brain surgery and would not consider it without very careful consideration. The rare incidence of my condition also means, rightfully so, that not every health care professional you meet will immediately understand what it is and the impact of it. It seems that a lot of people are diagnosed with a colloid cyst because they are presenting with symptoms such as headaches or migraines, vertigo, imbalance and many other symptoms, but we are told that the symptoms have nothing to do with the colloid cyst. So we spend the remainder of time after our diagnosis trying to quell any fears that the migraine or vertigo attack we have today could be related to our colloid cyst. We may head off to ER but get told the same thing: *It has nothing to do with your cyst.* Sometimes CT scans or MRIs are done—the images may be perfect except for that circular mass in the third ventricle of our brain. And so we carry on.

At least, that's how it was for me. They said my vertigo and other symptoms were not related to my colloid cyst. I had to learn to be okay with a migraine and not panic that it meant something more serious. This was sometimes hard to do, especially when it did not abate quickly. Looking back on the development of my hydrocephalus, the vertigo attack was prolonged. The migraine that lasted for nine days without any relief from a variety of medications, including IV medications, was vastly different from any migraine I had ever had before. But even the medical specialists in the referral hospital did not pick it up. The best lesson I learned from that experience is to keep being your own advocate. Unfortunately, this means that you may feel like a hypochondriac, and might even be treated as such. But ultimately it is your body and your life.

Because a colloid cyst is rare and there is not much scientific research into its effect on the brain, on the myriad of symptoms arising from the cyst, or on post-operative recovery of individuals with colloid cysts, it is hard to know what to expect. For the first time, I think about putting my experience down on paper. I know someone out there will have been diagnosed with a colloid cyst and be searching for answers. Maybe my journey will bolster someone else's courage.

I know that I have been affected by not having a definitive link between my cyst and the symptoms that suddenly appeared. This has impacted how I know my body, what I trust and what I don't trust, and whom I trust and don't trust in the medical system. I am more skeptical than I ever was of diagnosis and treatment. However, I do understand and support the fact that money and research needs to go to the majority of disease conditions. It does, however, leave some patients with little to grasp at.

One of the things I think that is hard for us as individuals who have been through brain surgery (and this applies to many other conditions) and feel 'terrible' is that we don't look sick. It is often more of an internal manifestation of fatigue, vertigo, dizziness, imbalance, memory loss and much more. Recently, someone asked how I was feeling. I said I was not feeling so great that day, especially after just having been back in hospital again, and they replied, "Well, you can at least be grateful that you are here."

And I am. I do not take one day for granted any more, I don't kiss my son goodnight without thinking what a miracle he is, and there are times I look at my husband and love him even more. But it is okay to for me to, yes, feel blessed, but also to feel ticked off and not so great sometimes because of what I've been through.

I have learned through this process that everyone has a unique life and experience. I judge people less on things they say or do, as I know that everything has an explanation or a meaning in our lives. We often don't know what is really going on behind everyone's faces and the masks they wear in society. I have more empathy for the people around me, especially those who may have 'invisible' conditions, such as a brain tumor, cancer, multiple sclerosis or even a mental health condition. Just because it's not as visible as a broken limb doesn't mean that it isn't serious.

I have been trying to see if there is any form of support group that I could attend for people in my own community who are recovering from brain surgery or a brain injury. However, I am struggling to find anything. I am able to walk, talk and basically function by myself. It is unfortunate that there is nothing for the in-between stage where you are trying to recover but at the same time need some extra guidance and help. I know the health care system dollars go towards the people who need them most and I totally agree with that. It would just be helpful if I could find something for the in-betweeners like me. The Facebook group is a fantastic resource, but I am looking for face-to-face contact. I will keep on seeing what I can find.

February 28

I am so tired of being so tired! I was so excited, as I had started back at gym and Pilates. I could feel my body craving the exercise and my movement-starved muscles loving the feel of moving again and being challenged, albeit at a tremendously-reduced level.

I had a busy Tuesday this week. Chiropractor, gym, haircut and hence did not nap, as it made no sense to come home for thirty minutes before fetching my son from school. I felt really good that day—so pleased with myself for doing it all, even at a much slower pace than I was used to. I thought missing just one nap could not be that bad; I am already six months post op!

Well, that has come tumbling down on me. Wednesday morning was okay but by the afternoon, I could feel the energy drain out of my body until, by 6:30 pm, I had to lie down. I had hit the wall that I had seen coming all day. And here I am on Thursday and have spent the entire day in bed as my body feels like a rag—my head's a bit dizzy but the fatigue is once again in every nerve and fiber of my being.

I feel like I climb these mountains and get so happy once I am near the top. But then I start feeling tired, and when I get to the 'top' I realize that I am nowhere near the real top of the mountain but have merely reached a small outcrop on the way up. I still have a long way to go.

The one lesson I am trying to learn, but it's a hard one, is to 'make time my friend and not my enemy.' By this, I mean trying to stop getting to the finish line as fast as I can. By making time my friend, I am taking some of the pressure off myself, by taking small steps each day instead of leaps, my chance of getting to the finish line is much higher. It is also the two steps forward one step backwards, right? Here's to hoping this is the way. My neurosurgeon's words come back to me about a one-year recovery. Maybe he was right. Give it time. I am only half way there.

Fourteen

MIND GAMES

March 1

I have started taking a picture of my favorite area on the seawall—
I am going to go back and take the same picture on the first day of
each month. This reminds me to take a breath and look at how
things have changed, improved or even perhaps not improved. Life
moves on; I want to take note of it, no matter how slow or fast it
seems to go. Take a moment to appreciate, and breathe.

What do my days look like at six - seven months post op?

My daily schedule at six months looks pretty much the same in that I
still have to nap each day. The difference is that I am now able to do a
little more exercise than I could do at four months. This is important
to my body and soul. My anemia is more under control as well, which
is helping my energy levels tremendously. I am still not able to work.
Given I am still napping, and still fatigued and highly reliant on a

tightly-controlled schedule to help keep the fatigue under control, now is not the time. It will come. Time is my friend and not my enemy.

March has arrived and the early signs of spring are coming. Buds peek out the soil and temperatures hit the double digits every so often— marvelous! I have just come back from my vestibular (balance) tests. That was quite an experience. It took about two hours to complete, with a list of instructions beforehand of what to do and what not to do. The worst part was the caloric testing, when they put these goggles on your eyes so all you see is darkness, then they pour warm water into your ears. Basically, this induces a vertigo attack. My worst nightmare. Then they have to do the other ear, too. Hang onto the chair and get ready for the ride.

After this testing I was finished; drove home and slept for two hours straight. I felt completely off kilter for the next two days, which makes sense given the onslaught my vestibular system was subjected to. It will be interesting to see what the test results will say.

In a magazine I found another thought, which was spoke to me today: *I may not be there yet, but I am closer than I was yesterday.* It is funny how the universe sometimes puts things in front of you just when you need them.

April 3

Spring is in full bloom—it is so beautiful and refreshing for the soul at this time of year. I feel as if one can watch the trees and flowers and actually see them grow. Being from the southern hemisphere, I still find the dramatic seasonal changes a novelty. The change in color and downfall of leaves in the fall, the new buds peeking out the soil in the beginning of spring, turning into the most beautiful bright-yellow tulips, cherry blossoms and so much more. I can almost feel my body trying to change along with the seasons.

I am now eight months post-op. I might consider myself the tulip bulb trying to bloom; behind the other bulbs that are already blooming, but determined to get out there and show its colors.

The results from my balance tests have come back. They show a balance system deficit and it says one of the tests may be suggestive of Superior Semi-circular Canal Dehiscence Syndrome (SSCDS), whatever that is.[18] But my ENT states that there is really nothing to worry about and that I should just keep active. If I feel it's necessary he could refer me to the balance clinic for further treatment, but the referral wait is quite long.

So, after finding that I am battling to walk around in the dark at night due to poor balance, I decide to do research of my own accord. I find that vestibular physiotherapy treatment can be useful for balance deficits. I locate a vestibular physiotherapist close to home and make an appointment. Hey, if I am going to bloom this spring, then it is best I get going!

April 18

The vestibular physiotherapist's approach is really interesting. She agrees that my current inability to walk around in the dark without taking out half the bedroom with me, as well as the previous vertigo attacks I have experienced, mean I should benefit from vestibular exercises. The exercises are based on movements that make me dizzy, which are done in order to train my brain to 'overlook the error messages' as a result of my balance deficit and carry on regardless. So, I commit to doing my daily vestibular exercises and see her every two weeks to assess my progress and get new exercises. An example of one of the exercises would be looking at an object but turning your head at a steady pace from side to side while staring at the object until you

18 Superior Semi-circular Canal Dehiscence Syndrome (SSCDS) is a very rare medical condition where a thinning or complete absence of a portion of the temporal bone overlying the superior semicircular canal of the inner ear causes hypersensitivity to sound and balance disorders. http://www.californiaearinstitute.com/ear-disorders-semi-circular-california-ear-institute.php

start to feel dizzy. Then stop. She sees a lot of patients who have had some form of neurological or neurosurgical trauma. I feel like this is a step in the right direction.

What do my days look like at eight months post op?

I cannot believe that I am now eight months post op. Some days it feels like an eternity since the thirty-first of August and some days it feels like yesterday. The same for my body. Some days I feel almost 70 percent recovered, other days I feel only 30 percent recovered. I am still napping every day after lunch and fall dead asleep, and still knock off eight to nine solid hours at night. I am able to do my Pilates, but my other gym is hard on my body. My confidence has taken a knock over the past months, and emotionally I still feel fragile. I feel like my short term memory is improving but I still use lists to keep track of my things to do for the day.

May 28

Today I quit my personal training, for the time being, anyway, until I can get my energy levels back. I was so enjoying it and could feel my body responding.

But my energy is so fractured at the moment that I still need to be vigilant each day. So until I get on a more even keel, I will focus on walking and doing my Pilates. I have got to do something for my core, which is still weak in general and pocketed with fat from the dexamethasone. I continue seeing my vestibular physiotherapist every two weeks or so and progress with the exercises and modifications that she makes. I can say that I am feeling progress with them. One of my main challenges was going to the bathroom at night and feeling completely disorientated, I feel a small improvement, but Rome was not built in a day. I will persevere.

After chatting to two of my best friends who have both—either currently or in the past—sought some advice and help from a clinical therapist or psychologist, I make an appointment to see a local woman, Sophia, who is South African and apparently really great. Not quite sure what to expect. Am I going to lie down on a couch and reveal all my deep dark secrets? After doing my research, I know that elevated cortisol levels can result in mood swings and even depression and I don't want to head down that road. I also need some help in figuring out and learning how to deal with my fractured energy levels, the ups and downs of my recovery, and my inability to commit to something without being concerned if my body can handle it. Because I am used to burning the candle whenever a job needs to be done, having the mental and physical stamina to carry on regardless.... this has been a learning curve of the greatest magnitude. So I think the time has come to speak to someone about all these thoughts.

Quite frankly, I am sure it would be boring for friends and family to hear what goes through my mind sometimes. Maybe they would think that I am lucky to be alive and not have to work immediately, so I should just enjoy it. But in my mind it is not working out that way. Believe me, it does not mean that I don't realize how blessed I am in the way things turned out, the supportive husband and family I have, and friends as well, but I do feel the need for some objective advice.

At first I found it strange to visit a psychologist, having not done this before. But after a while, I felt more at ease. Sophia explained that any trauma to the brain, whether from the hydrocephalus or the surgery, in my case, could impact areas of the brain that affect hormones and emotions.

After going over my story and current situation, she hit the nail on the head. "Your body and brain still feel like they are in a stress response mode."

This could explain my heavy fatigue, my altered hormone levels and my inability to continue with certain physical things such as gym, as it was too much stress on my body. It was a posttraumatic stress response that my body was still going through from the trauma of getting ill, being misdiagnosed, flying out of country for surgery and then having surgery.

Now I am in the right place to help my brain deal with what happened to it and to realize that it is now safe and can stop fighting. My one take-home idea was to try and start meditating to help my brain to 'zone out' of its high stress mode, allowing it to come down a level and start to calm down. For this, she recommended I listen to the highly-regarded Jon Kabat-Zinn, Professor of Medicine Emeritus and founding director of the Stress Reduction Clinic and the Center for Mindfulness in Medicine, Health Care, and Society at the University of Massachusetts Medical School.

I purchased an app online for my phone and started listening to his words before napping, and found I slept a lot deeper and woke more rested. Namaste! A key message in one of his meditations was to make sure you live in the present, and not on autopilot. "When you are in the shower, really be in the shower!" I thought that was great advice, as we so often go on autopilot through many of our day-to-day chores. There could instead be moments in which we could relax, enjoy and think, and get so much more out of them than we do.

One of the things Sophia and I also discussed was my decreased level of confidence. This has improved markedly, but was very difficult in the earlier days post surgery. She said it made sense given everything I had been through, and given the fact that as well as the trauma to my brain, I had to relinquish control over many aspects of my life.

On a side note, the survey we did on post-op patients in our Colloid Cyst Survivors Facebook group showed that over 50 percent experienced a lack of confidence in their first year post op along with high levels of 'slow thinking' and cognitive issues, short-term memory loss and fatigue. These were all issues I had personally faced. Of course fatigue, slow thinking and short-term memory loss would make self-confidence a challenge to anyone.

She also explained that my brain was almost like an infant brain at this stage. It needed to be protected during its recovery, and many things would over-stimulate it that would have not done so before. This made sense to me, as I found so many things were too much for me now. Too much noise, too much light, too many people around, and my brain started to protest and shut down. Just like Aiden, when he was an infant: too much stimulation and he would start to protest.

These visits to my psychologist are all starting to make sense, like putting a puzzle together and seeing the picture slowly start to emerge. I wish I had known about therapy earlier.

June 5

On my way back from dropping Aiden at school, I listen to the radio announcer comment on a study that found a connection between a lack of sleep in women and the success of their marriages. Women battle to fall asleep as quickly as men do, and hence often wake up crankier, more critical and shorter tempered than their spouses.

I can relate to that feeling, even though I am actually getting enough sleep at night and my marriage is in good nick. My husband calls a spade a spade. He commented to me last night that by the evenings I am often short-tempered and harsh with Aiden. My first reaction was to get defensive, but deep down I knew immediately that he was right. It often takes the person closest to you to make a comment that is completely honest, as difficult as it might be to take it on board.

The combination of heavy fatigue and the end-of-day antics from my strong-willed six-year-old sometimes leaves me feeling like a walking skeleton. I have had the biggest lesson in what fatigue does to you as a person, how it can chip away at your personality until at times you do not recognize yourself. The ability to be rational, see things in perspective and see the humorous side of things is often lost in a sea of mugginess. Things are remarkably better than they were after my surgery but still, almost ten months post-surgery, I need to nap each day. Some evenings I feel more exhausted than others. But maybe I have also got into the habit of being short-tempered as well. I am going to try to be more aware of myself, my comments and try to get back to enjoying the free-spirited nature of a six-year-old instead of it feeling like it's an energy drainer. My husband was spot on... again.

My short-term memory is still not what is used to be, but nothing that cannot be blamed on old age, I think. The other day when shopping with my son I needed to get a new shopping basket as our shopping was piling up. Of course I could not for the life of me remember what the name was for the shopping basket—I stood staring at it blankly until eventually Aiden said, "Don't worry, Mom, just call it thingam-ajig." And so from now on, all items whose names disappear at the opportune moment will be named thingamajig! He has also told me that I have the memory of a goldfish, so there you have it.

I have just been reading up on my neurosurgeon, Dr. Q's, website at Johns Hopkins. Every so often I do this to remind myself of how lucky I am. I am truly reminded this time around. I have been reading the blog of a brain cancer patient of Dr. Q's. He was not as lucky as I, although he battled like a warrior. I remember that after I had brain surgery, I thanked God that I did not have brain cancer and have the trauma of enduring surgery and then relentless treatments of chemotherapy or radiation. For me, brain surgery was hard enough.

I then realized that this is only the beginning for a lot of people who still have months of treatment ahead of them, and unanswered questions, while they are still trying to recover from intrusive brain surgery. Dr. Q raises money with fellow team members and even patients of his towards finding a cure for brain cancer. They do this through a variety of fundraisers but also through running in various races. They have coined a motto for their race t-shirts: "Inside all of us is hope." What a great phrase, and so true.

When we came home from Baltimore I donated my gran's inheritance money to Dr. Q's fund for finding a cure for brain cancer. He is such a motivational individual who has true compassion for his patients and I felt that this money would be in good hands. He continues to fundraise, goes to Washington to ask for more money for research into brain cancer and still manages to be a dad and husband. I made a pact with myself when in ICU that when I was able to, I was going to do something that made a difference and helped others. The August before I got sick I had been working hard on a business plan to help people less fortunate, to empower people who had never had that feeling of empowerment. After the brain surgery, lying alone in the ICU in the still of the night had brought this feeling of powerlessness home with a thud.

Although I am taking a break from working on my business plan to focus on a full recovery, I know that this is my future. I know this too, when I read other people's stories that have not ended positively, that I want to work each day—yes, to have a salary, but more importantly to know that my end impact reaches further than just me—that it reaches people for whom it makes a measurable difference.

June 13

I have had such a great two weeks; my energy is much better and I am starting to feel 'normal.' I think I have realized that I am just going to need to find my new normal. I am not sure what that is, what it looks like—but I think it is going to be better for me all round.

However, as good as I feel now, I can also feel the wall coming. I wake up and my body is slow, my legs ache, my head is slightly dizzy and I am exhausted. On Tuesday I did not nap, as I had my neurologist follow-up, and yesterday my son had a play date which was extremely noisy with lots of joyful screaming—that drains me so quickly. My face is numb and I can feel the life drain out of me. I am hopeful that my appointment today with the endocrinologist will shed some light on this issue.

As I sit in the endocrinologist's office, I am not sure what to feel. She has basically said that she sees no issues with my elevated cortisol levels, anemia and the symptoms I have described to her. I was hoping that maybe she would give me the silver-bullet analysis and say absolutely; your symptoms are a result of the elevated cortisol and other hormones. It is hard, as I have been scouring the Internet, which I realize has its pros and cons, and from what I have read, my symptoms might be attributed to the hormones. But I don't have the specialist training in this area, so I cannot honestly say that I know the ins and outs.

So, I think I will have my MRI in August, see my neurosurgeon and if nothing is resolving, I will ask my neurosurgeon for help and guidance. I do feel overall like I am still climbing upwards, I am on a positive slope but the slide-backs are still there. This time it was two weeks of feeling good before I hit the wall. At least the time frames between the slides backwards are getting longer.

The endocrinologist also says the same thing my local neurosurgeon said: give yourself a year to recover, then reassess. Fair enough. Once again, I realize I am lucky I don't have to rush back to work right now, as I just could not do it. How would I work when I need to nap? And some days are very low energy and would not be conducive to working on strategic direction or a complicated timeline.

June 14

Even though I hit a wall yesterday, I feel better today. I am keeping track of things like this; it helps me feel like I am making progress!

My 'hit the wall' symptoms are:

- Fatigue, at first mild then progressing to overwhelming

- Feel like the life is draining out of me

- Numb feeling starting in face and then moving through body

- Dizzy feeling

- Migraine/headache

Yes, I still get migraines. I thought they would have done a disappearing act with the removal of my in-house resident, the colloid cyst. But, for whatever reason, the migraines are here to stay. They started when the cyst was diagnosed at the size of 1 centimeter and maybe it is related and maybe it is not, but if that is all I have to be left with after my surgery so be it. *(Out of interest, when we conducted a survey of our Facebook group, over 50 percent of post-surgical members suffered from headaches or migraines in the first year post-operatively.)*

My vestibular physiotherapist is still helping me with my symptoms, especially my 'hit-the-wall' symptoms. She tests me at every visit to see how I am progressing and notices a marked improvement. I notice this in day-to-day life as well. This is what I wanted, a tangible improvement in my day-to-day life. I am not talking about things that impact people around me, but things that I notice on a small level that impact me alone.

I saw my psychologist again today. There is something refreshing about taking the more scenic route when I visit her. For once, things are not about blood tests, MRI results and surgical outcomes. We focus on how to help me, as a brain tumor and brain surgery survivor, manage my recovery. Some of the key things I learned today from Sophia: make special time each day for Aiden. This will help build a strong connection between us and build up the positive memory bank. Aiden needs quality time with his mom when she is not exhausted and ratty, so this needs to take place straight after school or in the morning, not at the end of the day. It will help me feel better as a mom so I will not feel so guilty that I am only sending out negative and frustrated vibes by the end of the day.

We also talked about how I am going to manage the summer. Ten long weeks of 24/7 momship await me. I am not too worried about it as I have Aiden in a few summer camps, the rush of the early morning will no longer be an issue, and I have a great babysitter I am going to call in once or twice a week to give me some space.

She also reiterated the importance of continuing my meditation. The first time I did it, I napped directly after fifteen minutes of meditation. I went to sleep and was out stone cold and woke up with a sense of "wow, what was that?"

Over the past months I have also become very in tune with my body and the triggers that drain my energy

The triggers that leave me feeling off-kilter are:

- Not enough sleep (less than 8 hours at night!), cutting naps or going to sleep too late;

- Too much noise—I can almost feel my energy draining out my body when exposed to lots of noise continuously, e.g. being at a kids' play gym indoors for more than an hour leaves me finished;

- Too many people or things going on around me—My brain needs to have more quiet time than active 'go-get-it" time at the moment. I now plan around this. It does not mean I don't go to a big party; it means I might not stay till the bitter end;

- Too much going on—Ha, big life moment for me. I check my daily and weekly calendar on a regular basis to ensure that my diary does not get inundated with 'things to do! I push things out to another, less-busy day if I need to.

By interacting with different health care professionals, I have gained insights from them all. My vestibular therapist pointed out to me today that I am imprinting in my mind and the way I think about things before I even do it. For example, standing on my 'bad' leg, I anticipate that the task will be more challenging for me than if I were standing on my 'good' leg.

It makes a lot of sense. I have not normally been scared of trying new things or being hindered by my own inability. But the past couple of years have taken their toll on me, physically, to the extent that I am more cautious than I was before. I subconsciously and consciously think things through before doing them. This might also be because I am now a mom; that changes things.

Note to self: within the realm of being sensible, try things out that perhaps were not so great for me before and see what happens. I might just be surprised. Also, don't set my body up by pre-conditioning it in my mind as to what my abilities are from past experiences. I'm going to try this out and see how it works.

Fifteen

FINDING INSPIRATIONS

June 18

This has been on my mind for a while: how can I give back and raise money for brain tumor research without jeopardizing my recovery? I am coming up to one-year post brain surgery on the thirty-first of August. I was thinking of doing a five-kilometer walk and raising money for Dr. Q and his research. I don't really have the energy to walk more than about five kilometers, and that would be walking. At the same time, I will look around for other five-kilometer walks in Vancouver that raise money for causes close to my heart. This will be a good thing to do mentally, emotionally and physically. I am going to see if I can get some friends and my family to join me in the walk. Start small.

People have asked me if it feels like 'one step forwards, two steps backwards' during my recovery from brain surgery. Even on a day where my energy tank is low and I am not feeling great, I know that this journey is more like '*two steps forward, one step back*' for me. The back steps have been hard; there is no joking about that. So, I have decided to call my fundraising effort Two Steps Forward. When you feel like you are just starting to get there, your body and brain teaches you otherwise; they pull you over and give you a speeding ticket. As frustrating as that is, I know I am heading in the right direction, which is the road to recovery. I have no idea how long that will take to be honest, not sure what the "new normal" is for me, but I know it is all in a positive direction, the right direction. Two Steps forward it is!

I had another great session with Sophia today. Why I did not start therapy earlier, who knows. All I know now is that if you feel the need to see a therapist or psychologist, just do it. Especially if you have suffered from any brain injury, concussion or brain surgery.

Today we discussed my actual surgery. She said that she noticed it was very hard for me to talk about the surgery and events leading up to it. She noticed I started to tear up immediately. This was so true. During the first months after surgery I relived the few days and hours before and after my surgery every day in my mind. Every time I closed my eyes to sleep something would surface, whether it was the sound of all the ICU equipment, or the MRI machine, or the OR nurse holding my hand as I went under.

Given the traumatic nature of the events leading up to my surgery, it was like a movie reel stuck in my mind on replay. She explained the difference between the prefrontal cortex of the brain and the amygdala. The amygdala is the part of the brain that would have dealt with the fear and survival mechanism evoked in my brain before surgery. It regulates and blocks information from going to your prefrontal cortex and this allows you to react quickly in a fight, flight or freeze situation. The prefrontal cortex is the 'wise leader' of the brain, which uses all the important information around us to help focus, analyze, reason and decide what is going on.

In a stressful situation or with post-traumatic stress, it is as if the amygdala is still switched on in fight, flight or freeze mode. Hence, the prefrontal cortex is not getting all the information it needs to think clearly. She asked me if I remembered the first time I acknowledged that I had survived after the surgery. I remember it as clear as day. It was the second night post surgery and I was in my ICU bed, joined by the many beeps and noises of the machines next to me. My head was bandaged and I was unable to move much due to the IV lines crossing my body. I remember thinking, "I am blessed, I have made it, and I will do something good with my life when I am able, I will learn from this and use it to do something I can look back on with strength."

Since my surgery, every time I close my eyes I say the Lord's Prayer, and I say that am blessed to be alive, and say my thanks for the list of people I am grateful for. I am not an overly religious person; I do believe there is something greater than just the human race, but for me it revolves more around the compassion of mankind and the ability to do unto others as you would like to be done unto you.

She suggests adding a couple more phrases to my 'prayers' at night: "You have survived, you are safe and you are protected." This will allow my amygdala to start calming down, allow it to realize that I am no longer in survival mode. I am a survivor.

This all made sense to me. In fact, one of the action steps in the pamphlet, *Brain Tumors and Fatigue* (issued by The Preston Robert Tisch Brain Tumor Center) states: Are you in survival mode or recovery mode?" My body, in many ways, has been stuck in survival mode. It will take time for my body to realize that it is no longer required to fight. It can relax. It has survived. We survived.

Interesting lesson: this can be seen in people who suffer from post-traumatic stress disorder (PTSD)—their body still functions in survival mode. I wish it were as easy as flicking a light switch on and off to change modes, but then I suppose the lessons we learn from these experiences would not exist. I think this is an important part of post-surgical care for many patients recovering from brain surgery, especially emergency surgery. For patients suffering from colloid cysts, they might not even know that they have the colloid cyst, or they might know they have the colloid cyst but suddenly develop hydrocephalus and require emergency surgery. Both of these situations do not allow the patient to mentally prepare for brain surgery and the emotional perspective that comes with it.

So, the physical recovery is one issue to deal with, but there is mental and emotional recovery as well, especially when you have had your brain worked on, the center of your emotional and mental health. I wonder how often this is acknowledged as an area that requires post-surgical treatment or rehabilitation? A post-traumatic stress response might not show up immediately after surgery, either. This is something for patients and caregivers to be mindful of, and they should speak to their health care provider about if they feel it is necessary.

Therapy has been a necessary part of my recovery. I should have done it earlier, but better late than never. Everything I learned in those sessions with my psychologist still helps me today in my daily life.

June 21

It is the last day of school today then the kids are unleashed on us for ten weeks of holidays. I have planned out the holidays with a few summer camps, two mini-vacations away to local areas as a family, and help from our babysitter who is home for the holidays. I am actually looking forward to it with a healthy dose of trepidation. Aiden is used to me having to nap on the weekends, so we have chatted about the fact that mom still needs to nap each day in order for the rest of the day to continue normally. My body is summer-ready: ten months post op and short-term memory much improved, fatigue getting better, confidence much improved and anemia resolved. I have still not returned to work. My body is not quite ready, but I hope to reassess the situation with my GP and my body by the end of summer.

I have come almost full circle now. Before, when I thought of what things would look like one year after brain surgery, I struggled to think that far ahead. When my neurosurgeon told me about the one-year recovery that was a hard line for me to accept, but it was oh so true.

What do things look like as I approach this line in the sand? I am still affected by my surgery but I'm leaps and bounds ahead of where I came from. I am still easily fatigued but way stronger than I was. I battle with noise, lights, and too much going on, but have learned strategies to cope with these and place less blame on myself for having days where I feel like a failure. I am still often 'monster mom' at the end of the day, but am more aware of my impatience and its relation to my fatigue, and I make sure each day that I connect with Aiden on a positive level.

I may look and act exactly the same as I used to prior to surgery, but I am changed. In a positive way, in a stronger way. I have survived. And that is the most important part of all.

July 1

The Facebook Colloid Cyst Survivors group I belong to is amazing. There are now over 720 members, and so many different stories. I often go there with questions of my own or just to learn from other peoples' experiences and outcomes or to give support. It has been so useful to ask questions when I am feeling low, or when I have issues with my energy levels. It helps to hear I am not alone and I am not being weird and that yes, it is frustrating that this is happening. It truly is the people who have the same condition or have had brain surgery who understand what both the pre- and post-op situations feel like.

Previously a couple of group members had conducted a survey relevant to pre and post surgery. I asked the group founder if I could put together more questions based on the original survey, plus questions and topics that have come up in the group, and also questions I think would be interesting to both colloid cyst sufferers and health care professionals. Given the experience I have had with my colloid cyst and pre-surgical misdiagnosis, any way I can get more information out there, the better. So, I have set up a survey on surveymonkey.com so we can analyze and get the results in various formats. It will be interesting to see how many respondents we can get and what the outcomes will be. Examples of some of the questions are: At what age did you start suffering from headaches leading up to diagnosis, what size was your colloid cyst upon diagnosis, how long did it take from diagnosis to surgery, and questions on symptoms profile as well.

After the first week we have over 100 respondents to the survey—this is fantastic! I have compiled the results into a PDF document that everyone can read and even take to their neurosurgeon if they want.

July 22

Two weeks later and we have hit the 200 mark! Two hundred members of the group have responded, and the information is very interesting! I have also compiled extra questions that we could pose in the future, with cross-analysis with the data e.g. at what size did the colloid cyst result in hydrocephalus, at what size did the colloid cyst result in enough symptoms to warrant surgery?

I wonder whether this information could be taken further. All the scientific studies out there on colloid cysts are of smaller group sizes, or are focusing on the surgical technique and not necessarily patient experiences or quality of life. My shooting-star wish would be to get this data worked on and published in the right format in a medical journal of sorts. Imagine that! Somewhere where people suffering from a colloid cyst can access the information when they are looking for it and where medical professionals can discover and learn more about the pre- and post-op experience from a colloid cyst patient's perspective. Let's wait and see.

August 7

It is time for my almost-one-year MRI. Lying in that all too familiar MRI tube, I realize it is my ninth brain MRI in three years. Although I felt a little apprehensive about it, as I did when I still had the cyst, I now know that I cannot change what will happen in the future, it will be what it will be. And we will get through it; the good, the bad and the ugly.

August 19

Today is an important day. It is my one-year follow up with my neuro-surgeon here in Vancouver. The amazing news is my MRI is all clear. What a sigh of relief. In a nutshell, my other symptoms of short-term memory challenges, confidence and fatigue should only get better as the next year comes around. Now I am happy to wait another year. I have just had the hardest year of my life, and I now know I can do it.

When I saw the neurosurgeon last time, just after my surgery, he told me to wait one year before I would feel like I had not had brain surgery. That seemed like an eternity, but here it is. I have tears of happiness in my eyes, knowing this past year has taught me so much about myself, my family and my body, and about life in general. I now know that what comes around the corner is not predictable but the best I can do is take it one day at a time.

I am also now at the stage that I don't link each and every issue I have to my brain surgery. It could just be something that might happen to anyone, e.g. migraines, short-term memory issues. This is a step forward and I think also helps with my whole recovery process. I also think this stage happens only with time; in the acute recovery stage it is not as easy to dismiss symptoms.

Another reminder of how things have changed over the past year, if not the past months, is my confidence. It is certainly not near where it was before my surgery, but it is markedly improved. And as my neurosurgeon said, the next year I will just continue to see improvements - Looking forward to the next year!

Sixteen

BRAINIVERSARY

August 27

Summer already seems to be passing us by. It has been a good summer. Aiden and I have spent many days in the sun with friends, and days with just the two of us. He has been really good at knowing when I need to nap and good at entertaining himself when needed. I can feel my body is gearing up to stop naps. This is going to be amazing, not having to plan my life around being at home after lunch. I am looking forward to this next step.

Aiden and I had a chat today about the importance of wearing a helmet when doing any activities and sports that require it. I just wanted to get this off my chest, as a concussion can also have a dramatic effect on a person's life. Having been through the past year, I have come to appreciate how amazing one's brain is and, at the same time, how very important it is to protect it whenever it is vulnerable. I don't mean wearing a helmet at all times. But even a short ride on a scooter at a friend's house could be the one time you don't wear a helmet and the one time you fall. Aiden understands that it is his body to look after and he needs to know how important his brain is to him and to us.

He asks, "what if they don't have a helmet?"

I say that it's his body, and no one can force him to go on a scooter without a helmet. He needs to say "no, I will not do it without a helmet, as I could hurt my brain".

The time has also come for me to do something concrete about the journey I have taken this past year. I have been inspired by many people who belong to the Colloid Cyst Survivors Facebook group, as well as by general stories in the community about people with brain tumors and brain cancer. Now that my energy is returning, I have decided to start my fundraising. Firstly for the Brain Tumour Foundation of Canada, and secondly for Dr. Q. I strongly want to support a local charity but at the same time, I have the utmost gratitude and respect for the work that Dr. Q is doing. So, let's see how this goes.

I already have the name chosen, Two Steps Forward, so I set up my website for fundraising, join the donation networks for the two causes, and send out emails to all my friends and family letting them know what I plan to do. I am going to start off slow and do two five-kilometer walks: one on my brainiversary, the thirty-first of August, and the next an organized five-kilometer walk/run event in Vancouver. In our survivor group we call it our brainiversary: the day that commemorates when we had surgery. We celebrate as each group member passes this milestone. Thereafter for my fundraising, I will plan an activity each month to raise funds. I have set my goals and hope that I can over-achieve. I know it may not seem that large a goal, but I firmly believe that every dollar helps.

The colloid cyst survey is going well and we now have over 260 respondents! I decide that the time has come to send the study to Dr. Q. I would really like his input on whether this information is worth taking further. How can the data be used to benefit both patients and medical professionals?

I am super excited, over the moon, when I get an email back from Dr. Q saying that he and his team would be interested in seeing if we can work together on it and look at getting it published in a top neurosurgical journal. Imagine how fantastic that would be! Given the incidence of colloid cysts at 3 per million, our 260+ survey respondents cover a population of 250 million.

I have to modify the survey for Johns Hopkins with some additional questions, which will allow for more objective analysis of headaches and quality of life. People will need to do the survey again but in the interests of getting this information out and published, I am hoping this will not be a big issue. The Johns Hopkins team and Dr. Chaichana, a colleague of Dr. Q's, have been so helpful and positive about getting this done! This effort also helps me on an emotional level. Th more information out there, the less chance of misdiagnosis happening to someone else.

August 31

Today is the day. I wake up in my own bed and can honestly say that I feel blessed. Yesterday I was feeling a bit emotional over the realization that exactly one year ago I was in my ICU bed awaiting brain surgery. But, this morning I feel like I have passed a milestone in my life. It feels so good, like a weight has been lifted. I think this is also largely due to my increased energy levels and sense of well-being that I have really noticed over the past few weeks.

Today marks the beginning of my fundraising efforts. We do our walk today and the weather could not have been more perfect—the sky is clear blue, the sun is warm and it's a perfect day to celebrate being here in this moment. I chose the seawall to start my fundraising as it has been an important stepping stone in my recovery, from those few steps I took in the beginning to being able to comfortably walk it several times a week and enjoy the scenery and fresh air. It has been a healthy contributor to my physical and mental health!

A group of close friends join us in the walk and the kids have a ball climbing rocks, walking the seawall and enjoying the weather afterwards at the impromptu picnic in the park. I could not have asked for a better start to my 'New Year!'

I think I have made peace with myself and what has happened, and what that actually means to me. It has taken some time and some work. In fact, a lot of work. Being active, on the go and juggling more than I can is an intrinsic part of who I am so this has not been an easy lesson.

But while it has been hard, it has been good for me. I am taking time to 'smell the roses', find a 'new' normal and really appreciate the journey we have all been through the past year. I cannot say that tomorrow will be joyful and full of activity for me. I realize that I can no longer predict what tomorrow will bring. But I can be positive about it. I can manage my life to minimize negative outcomes but I can also try new things—things that might have been a bad idea three months ago; with more stamina now, I can try them and see.

A huge lesson that I have taken out of this year is that some things matter and some just don't matter. I tend to get wrapped up in the day-to-day of life, the hustle and the bustle, and forget that we may only be here for a moment. Each day is precious; each experience, both good and bad, has some impact and relevance. I have realized that my family and friends are so very special. I knew this before, but now it is even more amplified. I also know that I want to make a difference, whether it is big or small, in case that moment passes by and my time here is complete. What will I leave behind? I have also learned to be in tune with my body. I respect its abilities, I know its boundaries but most of all I know what marvelous things our minds and bodies can achieve, especially in the face of adversity. Thank you for these lessons.

What do my days look like one year post surgery?

I am just about to stop napping every day after lunch. I can feel my body is almost ready to do so. Great relief. The difference at one year post op is huge. I feel almost 90 percent recovered. At the same time, I am mindful of my body and respectful of it and not overdoing it to the nth degree. I get the odd migraine but my medication seems to tackle it head on.

September 3

Today the decision arrived in the post from the College of Physicians and Surgeons of British Columbia regarding my complaint about my misdiagnosis in August. I open the envelope with a sense of trepidation.

The document is long and arduous to read, so I skip towards the end. In a nutshell, they found no issue with the conduct of the one neurol-ogist but put criticism on the younger neurologist, whom they stated should have taken more due care with imaging, given my medical history. There will be a permanent note on the neurologist's record and this will be a 'lesson' for the neurologist for the future. Pity I had to be the guinea pig.

However, I have achieved my main aim of ensuring that the situation was brought to the attention of the relevant medical board. Book closed and on the shelf, hopefully never to be opened again.

September 4

It is the end of a magical summer. Back to school for Aiden and back to reality for me. No more long summer days with endless hours. I remember my nervousness at the beginning of the summer holidays as I contemplated how I was going to manage looking after Aiden while in recovery mode.

But now it's September and I must admit, I do actually relish the thought of having my first cuppa coffee in the coffee shop along with the other moms, as we all sit in silence and take a deep breath. Peace and quiet for a moment in our lives.

This has been a healing summer for me. I have now thrown my daily naps out the door—yippee! My body is strong enough to get through the day without some shut-eye. I feel like a toddler shedding its skin.

September 12

Mid-September and it's thirty-one degrees Celsius here (almost ninety degrees Fahrenheit. After school, Aiden and I seize the kayak and spend the afternoon exploring coves and hovering over purple starfish and secret seaweed. Magical and cherished moments. An Indian summer.

September 17

Today I dressed up. I put on my high heels, smart pants and dress shirt and pulled out my 'work' jewelry from the mothballs. I am attending The Art of Marketing conference in the city. This is the first time I have got into 'work mode' since June last year. It feels fun to dress up, I feel like I am on a mission. Key objective: go and get up to speed with what is new in marketing. Use these lessons to benefit my work, but also my fundraising.

I had to laugh at Aiden. He has become so accustomed to me being at home since my surgery that when he saw me dressed up, it set off alarm bells in his head. His immediate response was: "You don't look good, Mom!" In other words: 'Hang on a moment, I am not sure I like seeing you in smart work clothes, this may mean you are going back to work. I am not sure I like this scenario.'

What a great morning: learning things again, being challenged and allowing my mind to explore new strategies and ways of thinking. I also have the opportunity to catch up with clients and past work colleagues, which is fantastic. I feel like I used to, over a year ago: back in the driver's seat. However, after three hours of lectures and focusing, my brain starts to slow down. I feel exhausted, the people around me are moving too fast and I am just too slow. Although this realization tells me I am not yet ready to return to work, this is a step in the right direction.

I am so glad I have done this today! I felt the adrenaline coursing through my veins in a good way.

Seventeen

TWO STEPS TO THE SIDE

September 23

It's drawing near to the end of September. Aiden is back at school and the summer is done and dusted. The strangest thing is that I have noticed that my fatigue is coming back. What? I am now getting so tired again by the end of the day. The 'mommy monster' is back by about 5 pm and she's not pretty.

I also notice that I feel slightly off balance, a similar feeling to what I experienced after my brain surgery. I ask my vestibular physiotherapist about this. I have only had three to four weeks' reprieve from napping and my body seems to not be coping very well at all. Perhaps I have over done it? But seriously, I am one year post op: enough is enough!

September 27

The imbalance and disequilibrium (feeling like I am on a boat) increase and I find the fatigue (and the mommy monster) is becoming overbearing. I now need to now nap again during the day in order to make it to the afternoon. Deja vu!

It dawns on me to look back over the results from the balance tests I had done back in March 2013 after the December 2012 vertigo attack. The one thing that jumps out at me from the results is: Cervical Vestibular Evoked Myogenic Potentials (cVEMPS: *reduced thresholds on the right with a signifiant response seen at 70 dB. This can be suggestive of semicircular canal dehiscence syndrome (SSCDS).*[19]

What on earth is that? I have never heard of that condition. I just remember my ENT dismissing my balance test results, saying that there was nothing of great importance and that I should just 'get on with life and be active.' I recall being a bit irritated by that statement and hence seeking out the vestibular physiotherapist of my own accord. The physiotherapy had worked incredibly well.

I will wait a little longer and see if the imbalance and fatigue go away. Maybe back to school has been just as exhausting for me as it has for Aiden.

October 1

Fall is here. Everywhere I look, the leaves are changing color. There is a freshness in the air that I love about this time of year.

But I feel like I am also falling. My disequilibrium has not gotten any better. In fact, I feel like I am on a boat all day. I am absolutely fine driving; in fact this is the one time I feel good, so much that I wonder if maybe I should just drive all day—change of career, perhaps?

I am also napping every day now, otherwise the wheels fall off in the afternoon. I am finding that my migraines are also returning on a

---

19 Superior Semi-circular Canal Dehiscence Syndrome (SSCDS) is a very rare medical condition where a thinning or complete absence of a portion of the temporal bone overlying the superior semicircular canal of the inner ear causes hypersensitivity to sound and balance disorders. http://www.californiaearinstitute.com/ear-disorders-semi-circular-california-ear-institute.php

more frequent basis than they used to, and my neck muscles are all seized up.

I have decided to take matters into my own hands as I am so keen to get my health back on track fast and furiously, and the waiting times locally to see a specialist are just too long. I have already been off work for over a year now, and really want to get back to reality. So we are going to Seattle, to a dizziness clinic that specializes in vestibular issues. I think this is the right move. Let's see what they have to say about my ears. Is it my ears, or my head?

October 4

The otolaryngologist (head and neck surgeon with a specialty in neuro-otology) at the dizziness clinic in Seattle feels that my symptoms are actually being caused by my migraines—who would have thought? Migraines masking an imbalance—but apparently he sees a lot of this. So he has started me on TOPAMAX, a preventative migraine medication to take daily. We will see if it stops the disequilibrium, as well as any migraines I am having. Secondly, he wants me to have a CT temporal bone scan to rule out SSCDS (*superior semi-circular canal dehiscence syndrome*), He is doubtful that I have this, so it is not urgent to get it done. I am also going to start on a special migraine diet. This will help identify any dietary triggers causing my supposed migraines.

I am willing to do anything to kick these symptoms out the door for a speedy exit. I also make an appointment to see my local neurologist about my migraines.

October 5

Two hundred eleven respondents to the revised colloid cyst survey that I have been working with the Johns Hopkins team on! I have downloaded the final data and sent it off to Johns Hopkins. Pressing the send button on an email never felt so good. It will feel even better if this data produces information that will be of use to both the medical professional and the patient. I really hope that it will help open the doors on rare conditions such as the colloid cyst, especially from a patient perspective and relating to their quality of life. Fingers crossed. I know it will not be an overnight process; it might take up to nine months or longer. But good things take time, right?

October 31

My neurologist appointment puts a spanner in the works as he doubts my symptoms are due to my migraines and suspects it is my ears. So I begin the all-too-familiar roundabout of medical opinions on another rare condition. I really should enter the lotto on a more regular basis, especially if I get diagnosed with SSCDS after having a colloid cyst. It would seem my chances of hitting the jackpot on rarities is high.

November 6

So, I head off for a CT temporal bone scan while continuing on the new preventative migraine medication. Interesting, the number of migraines I am having has definitely decreased but my disequilibrium has not changed at all. Happy on the migraine front for sure!

My CT scan comes back with a statement that takes me by surprise: "Suspicious for bilateral superior canal dehiscence". What! Oh my goodness. This must be a joke! I was hoping for at least a one-sided issue only, but to have it on both sides—seriously? Can I get a break on this?

I am not sure what to think. On the one side I feel slightly relieved that there may be a reason behind the way I am feeling, on the other side I feel unsettled, as I am thoroughly clueless about what this means.

November 15

So off we head down to Seattle again. The doctor reviews my CT scan and advises that the next step is to have a barrage of testing done, to confirm that the dehiscence is actually physiologic—which means that it is actually causing my symptoms. He reviewed the options for treatment of SSCDS. If the dehiscence is indeed physiologic and the patient is suffering from enough symptoms to disrupt quality of life, then surgery is recommended. I would at this point, put my hand up and say yes, my quality of life is definitely being affected and I will have the surgery, doctor. While I have done some minor reading up on the condition, I was not prepared for the reality of the word craniotomy.

The current treatment for SSCDS is a craniotomy, i.e. brain surgery. So within the space of eighteen months, my brain may get to make another debut to the surgeon's scalpel. The thought is mind numbing, to put it literally.

My tests are booked for December back in Seattle and in the mean-time, I try not to let the overwhelming thoughts and fear flood my body and mind.

November 20

We have cancelled our trip to South Africa this Christmas. We did this even before I went for my CT scan. The trip is long and arduous even when you are in good health, but given that I am heavily fatigued, napping daily and struggling with my equilibrium, the thought of travelling for thirty-eight hours across the globe has started to weigh heavily on my mind.

I discussed it with Marchand, and he said that the fact that it was even crossing my mind was enough reason to cancel it. It was heartbreaking to do this, as I have not seen my parents since my surgery last year and have not seen my brother and his family in over two years. But I know my body will struggle.

My symptoms are progressively getting worse, yet different at the same time.

- *24/7 disequilibrium.* The best way to describe disequilibrium is that I feel like I am on a boat all day, but not in a good way. Sometimes I feel nauseous. I also feel as if I am walking on a trampoline all day: soft and spongy on the ground.

- *Visual overload.* Shopping in supermarkets can be visually overwhelming for me. I walk in feeling okay and walk out feeling as if I have drunk a bottle of wine. Not sure what the cashiers think of me by the time I reach the check out. The connection between the visual and vestibular systems is so clear to me in these circumstances.

Working on the computer for too long is also a challenge, especially scrolling down a page. I now need my sunglasses on more than I ever used to, even on an overcast day.

- *Extreme fatigue* and having to nap each day. My brain feels like it needs the warm and comforting blanket of silence just to recover from daily activity.

- *Intolerance to noise.* Washing dishes sounds like an orchestra in my own kitchen; the rustle of a plastic bag sounds like firecrackers.

- *Autophony.* My own voice, after a while, sounds too loud in my own head. I feel I need to speak softer. Heaven forbid I should need to raise my voice, as that just makes my head explode and the boat rock even more. I can also hear my *neck joints move.* This started about five months ago when I was doing my vestibular exercises one day. I realized I could hear my neck joints moving against each other, which I had never heard before—it was a grating and very unnerving sound. How weird!

- *Tinnitus* in both ears. I have had tinnitus for over eight years, but it is definitely here to stay.

I have spent the past weeks as most parents have been: busy with school events as we head towards the festive season and the close of school for the two-week Christmas holidays. My naps once again stake a claim in the middle of my day. I struggle to attend Aiden's hockey games, as the noise level is just too high and I feel my brain shutting down in protest. I make modifications so that I can continue to be part of it all: sit at a different part of the rink to watch him, behind the glass instead of right at the rink. There's nothing new about this dynamic for me, but I want to be as much a part of his life as I can. He is seven-and-a-half years old now and for the past eighteen months of his life I have been inactive and unwell. I try my best to hide how I am feeling from him but sometimes my mask falls by the wayside and it is not possible; even he sees through me.

December 3

We head off to Seattle again and after being seen by the otolaryngol-ogist and having more balance tests done to show if the dehiscence is physiologic, he recommends that I have surgery.

Marchand and I look at each other with a sense of disbelief. We decide to get a second opinion to ensure this is the right way forward. After seeing the balance test results as well, I am not 100 percent convinced about the brain surgery recommendation.

I cannot lie when I say that I have mixed feelings about being diagnosed with SSCDS. I am relieved that we have finally found out what is causing my symptoms and that there is a treatment. At the same time, the thought of undergoing brain surgery yet again is distressing. I know this is a different type of brain surgery but it is still a craniotomy. It involves drilling into my skull, IV lines, surgery and ICU. It involves recovery, and after just completing one year of a hard recovery, this is not an easy thing to wrap my head around.

But I know I cannot continue feeling like this. The continuous dis-equilibrium, worse around loud noises, heavy fatigue, and feeling nauseous all day and all night. It is time to stop all of this and get back to when things felt right.

This is not a pity party by any means. I am just so ready to get back to life, get back to doing things and not feel limited by my physical ability to do so. I just want to be back to being able to be Claire—the mom, the wife and friend that I used to be. I will be, just with a few more holes in my head, it seems!

I try to organize a remote second opinion at Johns Hopkins and they recommend I come in person instead. Given that I may be about to undertake brain surgery for a second time, we decide it is worth the trip. My GP has put in a request for a local otolaryngologist appoint-ment but I have been told the wait time is eight to twelve months. There is no chance I could continue feeling this way for that length of time.

The earliest appointment I can get in Baltimore is twelfth of February, which seems a lifetime away, but it is with one of the world experts in this condition so I am willing to wait it out. We have Christmas in the meantime and I know that the days will pass by quickly.

Mentally, I will use this time to prepare for the possibility of brain surgery again. Physically, I will try and keep my body as mobile as I can. It is not so easy, given that I feel like I am walking on a trampoline all day, but I cycle at home on our stationary bike and do a few exercises to keep my body from falling apart. I know how important it is to keep moving.

Unfortunately, I have had to put a hold on my fundraising activities, which makes me feel really down. I was so excited and motivated about pursuing this in August, but I know that now I need to focus my energies on just getting through the day.

The time will come again when I can get back on track. It will. I am getting good at learning the lesson of one step backwards, two steps forwards. I just have to keep reminding myself.

Eighteen

Baltimore Beckons

January 12

Strange how things have a way of arriving in your life when you need them most. I came across a website project called 365grateful.com. This focuses on taking a picture every day of something in your life for which you are grateful. I think I have truly learned the gift and art of gratitude over the past year, and really connect with this idea especially now, when things are a bit rocky, a bit unstable. It is important to look for the small things each day for which I am grateful.

It starts with photographs of the swirls of paint that my son is mixing, to pieces of LEGO that Aiden and I build together, to crisp frost on leaves outside my front door. I decide to commit to this project for the year; not every day, if I cannot—that is not the aim. The aim is to look for and acknowledge the small things around me, for which I am truly grateful.

I have noticed a big change in my symptoms over the past four weeks or so. I feel like my chronic disequilibrium is still here, but maybe my brain has adjusted to it. It feels like it might have decreased a little. Is it because I am getting used to it? Who knows.

However, I am getting more sensitive to noise in a big way. Oh, this is bad. Aiden commented one day that I looked as if I wanted to be sick after going into Safeway for ten minutes. He got it completely. Even going clothes shopping is a no-go. Well, this could be a bonus situation for a while. On-line shopping only!

Another issue is talking on the phone or even FaceTiming on the computer. I have tried switching ears when I am on the cordless phone but now, about five or ten minutes into the conversation, I can feel my equilibrium start to get worse and I almost feel a shift in my balance. It sounds strange, but I feel the cotton wool in my head descend and start to fog out my brain. And the sound of my own voice is still too loud in my own head.

Long distance phone calls longer than five minutes prove challenging. I might try speakerphone next time, as holding the phone close to my ear is just too much. I've got to think outside the box, here. The box literally being my skull, I think!

Time is passing and it is almost time for me to head off to Baltimore to see the specialist there, whom I hope will give me more insight into what is going on and bring relief to the current state of affairs going on in my body.

February 10

As I sit in the Toronto airport waiting for my flight to Baltimore, I am not sure what I am feeling. The flight from Vancouver was fine. I wore 'noise cancelling' earphones the whole way and so the engine noise was not too insane inside my head. On the ascent I also tried special earplugs to see if it would prevent my ears from getting sore from the change in cabin pressure. I also took decongestant nose spray. My ears seemed fine.

In the Toronto airport, though, I am now feeling really tired and off-kilter. I've just spoken to Marchand on the phone, and that along with the noise has made me feel completely off balance and drained. The usual. At the same time, I am glad this day has come. I am so ready for this. It has been two months since I got my last opinion of "yes, you need surgery," but not decisive enough on which ear. My symptoms have just been getting worse and worse and I am ready to have surgery to correct this and get my life back.

I am feeling bad enough to want to have brain surgery again—yes! I want to run around in the playground with my son and hear him shout with joy as he jumps in the air, I want to do a quick grocery shop without feeling drunk, I want meet my best friend in a coffee shop without feeling off balance, I want to go the whole day without having to nap, I want to be able to go walking with my husband and out to dinner thereafter and not fear I will literally fall down from exhaustion. I know I am going to the place that will help me get these answers. I know we are all ready for a year without any health-related stress in our lives.

Arriving in Baltimore was quite nostalgic for me. I stayed in the same hotel we stayed in for my surgery. Everything looked the same. Even the smell of the coffee shop provoked an intense reaction in me. It literally brought tears to my eyes. I had not prepared myself for this part of the trip at all: the trip down memory lane.

It is winter now; so many things look completely different compared to the heat of summer last time we were here. The hotel terrace, where the umbrellas used to overlook the water and people used to have a drink in the sun, is all wrapped up from the cold. The swimming pool, where Aiden used to spend hours basking in the sun and swimming like a fish, is closed.

Wrapped up warmly, I take a walk along the waterfront to the book-shop that I know my Mom and Aiden used to visit. Along the way I see, for the first time, all the Baltimore settings in the pictures that my Mom took of Aiden that summer—all the places they visited together and connected together. It is so strange and nostalgic, but healing at the same time. Here I am, second time around, recovered from that surgery, and about to potentially undergo another one. I have come so far!

I can do this again. I feel strong. I walk past the bench that I clearly remember using as a break point each time Mom and I used to go on my daily strolls to keep me moving after my surgery. It is still there, waiting to offer a welcome reprieve to anyone needing it.

At the hotel coffee shop I drink a cup of Hong Kong tea in honor of my dear Mom. At one of our usual restaurants I eat dinner in honor of my family. I sink into a bubble bath using the hotel's L'Occitane soap I now use at home. Our senses are like doors to our hearts opening memories we often think we had forgotten.

I spend the morning sinking my teeth into writing in my journal. Something about being back in Baltimore invigorates a need and desire to get my words down into something more than just my journal; it sparks my passion to turn my words into a book.

It is a busy twenty-four hours, and worthwhile for so many personal reasons. I will be forever grateful for this time.

February 12

It is an early morning wakeup call and I am lying on the table for yet another CT scan; this time probably the highest-resolution scan available. The smell of the room brings back memories of my surgery—amazing how smells are so evocative. It brings back the smell of the oxygen mask...tears prick my eyelids. Two minutes and it is all done. Super quick and easy. Now to the doctor's rooms for a few very specific tests for SSCDS, then I meet with him for his diagnosis and recommendations.

During a lengthy and worthwhile meeting with the specialist, he lets me know that the results from the CT scan show 'bilateral superior canal thinning'. The tests they performed showed bilateral—perhaps left greater than right—conductive hyperacusis, but the VEMP tests (typically used for SSCDS testing) were normal. He says they could not rule out SSCDS as a culprit in my disequilibrium; however, vestibular migraines are more of a prime suspect given the many other factors taken into account. Therefore, surgery is not an option at this stage, as it would not necessarily provide me with any relief. He recommends tripling my preventative migraine medication over the next six weeks, continuing to follow the migraine diet and a variety of other steps, and then we will reassess.

I am not sure whether to cry or laugh. For the past two months, since my diagnosis and the recommendation of surgery in December, I have mentally prepared myself for brain surgery again, and now a complete swing-around. In a positive direction, yes, but this has taken me completely by surprise. I came here expecting a confirmation of the diagnosis and had a list of twenty-six questions on the surgery and three questions as a backup, if he disagreed with the diagnosis.

However, as we talk further, I feel a sense of relief flood my body. No brain surgery means a lot of things to me. As long as I am able to get relief from my symptoms, it means a big deal to my family and me. This is good news. This is great news!

And so, I will be monitored again in six to twelve months to ensure that the thinning has not progressed. Once again, my life lessons of 'one day at a time' and 'change is the only constant' ring loudly in my ears. I know from doing my research online that thinning of the bones can have symptoms that are as debilitating as if you had holes, but I am going to try everything we discussed today. And I'm also going to adhere very strictly to the migraine diet, before I go any other route. I am going to believe that these other options will provide me with the relief I need.

What was really interesting to discuss with the specialist was the vicious circle that he sees many patients with my symptom profile go through. They seem to do a back-and-forth dance between the neurologist and himself, trying to get to the source of their migraines and vestibular symptoms; the neurologists not often believing that migraines could be the source of vestibular manifestations. They are currently doing a study on the symptomology of vestibular migraines in order to shed more light on this exact fact. Interesting!

So the fact of the matter is that I could just have ongoing migraines that have morphed into 'attacking' my vestibular system, instead of more of the traditional headache-type migraine one typically thinks of. This could just be my thing to take forward with me; it could be a remnant from my cyst, my surgery. Or it might not be; who knows.

While dashing to the airport I tell Marchand the news of my doctor's visit. Due to an approaching snowstorm a state of emergency is closing in on Baltimore.

Marchand cannot believe the news either. I once again leave Johns Hopkins and Baltimore, hoping not to have to return for health reasons in the near future. This place has been so good to me and to us but for now, I need to leave. I would return for a holiday, yes, but not for health reasons. I hope.

Nineteen

New Beginnings

February 13

As I return home from my trip Aiden is at the front door, shouting in glee at the top of his voice "Mommy, Mommy," jumping up and down. He leaps into my arms for a huge hug. He is so excited that I do not have to have surgery again—bless him. Life is good.

I may need brain surgery again in the next year, the next two years, or I may never need it. But I am not going to let that stop me doing things. I am going to concentrate on taking small steps forward towards getting my body back on track, reducing my symptoms and loving my family, my friends and body for all it goes through, all it keeps on giving me and allowing me to do. Yes, it gives me challenges, but at the same time it gives me so much. It gives me life.

Once again, this experience—the past five months—has given me another moment to breathe and learn, learn my weaknesses and strengths, learn to be thankful for everything I have, learn to work with what I have and not with what I don't have. I am grateful. I am blessed.

March 15

We are all in for a treat. Mom and Dad have decided on the spur of the moment to fly over and spend spring break with us. We are over the moon! We are not going anywhere as I have not been well enough, and we had made no plans, not knowing if I was going to have just had surgery.

It is now over a month since my return from Johns Hopkins and I can slowly feel a change coming. I am on a military regime of my medication and migraine diet in all efforts to combat my disequilibrium once and for all.

Now that we know the hospital is not in our plans for the near future, we have booked to go to Hawaii the week after spring break is finished, once the schools are back in and things have calmed down. Our little family is well overdue for a break, some time away from Vancouver. We need to relax in the sun and heal together.

April 7

Our Hawaii trip was well timed. I was well enough to fly. My medication was working enough that I didn't have to nap during the day. The heat of the sun, smell of the sea, sound of the birds and crash of the waves helped restore our souls and our bodies from all the turmoil of the past few months.

Aiden had a wonderful time with a new-found buddy from California and spent hours swimming each day. The day his friend Alex left, he was devastated. All this pointed to the makings of a well-spent holiday for us all.

April 30

Back in Vancouver, the sea is calming, I feel like the storm is passing me by. The swell of the ocean is less than it used to be and the boat I am on is no longer in a constant 24/7 motion. My medication regime is working. I can happily say that the diagnosis of vestibular migraine was most likely spot on, given my body's response to the daily migraine medication. I have also been able to pinpoint the dietary items (caffeine, chocolate, nuts, alcohol that trigger my disequilibrium by following the migraine diet. When I started to add things back to my diet, it was very easy to identify what caused symptoms and now I know what to avoid.

I feel liberated. It has been two months since my Baltimore trip and increasing my medication and I am a new person. No longer am I bound by naps, crippling fatigue, and a constant disequilibrium. I still feel tired and get a sense of disequilibrium when I am overtired, too stressed or if I eat a trigger food.

My visit to Johns Hopkins was a godsend on so many levels. I might have been recovering from unnecessary brain surgery with no positive results. I am so very grateful.

I have even been able to return to limited work for the first time in almost two years. I feel part of the human race. This day has finally come. I knew it would. I am still keeping tabs on myself not to overdo things and try and run a marathon before doing the ten-kilometer run! But, I know that I am on the right track.

My specialist at Johns Hopkins has recommended that I continue on this medication for at least another six months before even trying to wean off it, and I absolutely agree with him, I am not up to changing anything at this stage.

When I first go back to work I feel nervous, worried that my brain may not be able to function in the same manner as before. But as I slowly start back with my same client, I realize it is like riding a bicycle. Before long I feel comfortable and confident in my abilities to deliver as a consultant. I do, however, notice that my brain reaches a 'max-out capacity' really early on, depending on what type of work I am doing.

When I overdo it I can feel my brain start to protest, almost like it is going to explode and melt down.

I think it is a matter of retraining my brain to get back into work mode, like when you have been on maternity leave or vacation. So, I am taking it really slowly with the number of hours I am doing each week. I need to protect it and nurture it as it grows back into itself and finds its feet again.

June 3

I have been able to experience some amazing moments over the past few months as my medication allows my body and brain to return to life. These moments I will cherish: going on my first bike ride in the forest with my son, who cheered me on from the sidelines like a coach when I made it all the way. Finishing off a presentation to my client and knowing that I did a good job of it. Getting through a day with two play dates, with kids all around, and not passing out with fatigue by the end of it. Going on date night with my husband and not counting the minutes till I could get back and go to sleep. Gardening outside in the sun, playing soccer, watching the kids play baseball and just being able to do it. The miracle of being able to do it. Pure magic!

It is only when these simple, basic things in life are taken away from you that you realize how incredibly important they are to your sense of wellbeing. As an adult who has had these things given back, I am all the more grateful for them. It is like being able to 'breathe in the small things in life' and really feel them.

June 15

I went to a women's personal growth and empowerment workshop this weekend with a friend of mine's company SPARK Creations. I realized, after much soul searching, that the time has come for me to 'repackage' my brain surgery baggage. A wise friend there passed on a quote from Lena Horne, which really changed my perspective on things dramatically. The quote was: "It's not the load that breaks you down, it's the way you carry it."

Everyone has baggage that we carry through our lives. It is what shapes us, what makes us and we can never really get rid of it, nor should we try. It is what makes us who we are. But it is like a backpack or suitcase and can be as cumbersome, uncomfortable and exhausting to carry. What we can do is reshape it, repackage it and move its contents around so it does not hinder us, or make our journey through life uncomfortable or tiresome, or hold us back.

I have realized that my 'brain surgery baggage' has been holding me back in certain areas and anchored me to a time in my life that was traumatic and desperate. I needed to go through that time; it was part of my recovery. But now I need to let it go and repackage that bag. Yes, I had a brain tumor and brain surgery and climbed my mountain of recovery, but now it is done. I need to let it go for my sake, for my son's sake and my husband's sake.

I wept many tears over this weekend. Tears of grief, tears of frustration for the person I feel I might have lost, tears of gratitude for my progress, my family and friends, and tears of happiness for so much more. And with each tear, I gently push the experience away from me. With kindness I say 'thank you, I have learned so much, but it is now time for me to move forward.'

I felt that the energy I was using, whether subconsciously or consciously, on the whole experience of my surgery and recovery could be used on other things. The past two years will always be part of my baggage, but now that bag feels lighter, more tightly packed and not so awkward for me to carry. My frustration with my energy levels and issues with vestibular migraines and health issues that seem to come and go post surgery may well continue, but I have refocused my energy toward embracing life and loving completely and living that purpose on a daily basis.

A wise friend suggested focusing on saying I was growing my energy instead of saying I was struggling with my energy. Just by saying that a few times, I felt better. The mind is strong, and it's an even stronger force on the body.

I worked hard over this weekend to discover my own personal values and purpose and here they are now on paper before me. Now I need to move them into my everyday life. My values are *Believe, love, be powerfully courageous and grateful*. My purpose is *to embrace life and love completely*. How simple these words may seem to those reading them from a distance, but how very powerful and resonating they are to me, the person who pulled them out of my soul.

Another area that was mentioned during this weekend was that perfectionism can actually be from a fear of failure, and it can be a blockage in many ways. This was a new idea for me. I have been a perfectionist my whole life. The more I think about it, the more it rings true.

Funny how things have a way of coming to you all at once. I was listening to CBC Radio and they had an interview with Katty Kay and Claire Shipman, two highly respected journalists and news anchors who have co-authored a book called *The Confidence Code*, which looks at the science and art of self-assurance—what women should know. I listened with great interest to their interview and took home a few key notes: many of us spend far too much time overthinking and overdoing things, which results in a lack of action. And we are scared to fail.

The key act of reading their book actually helped me continue to write this book. I was spending far too much time trying to perfect each sentence, to the detriment of actually doing anything about it. I was scared to fail. What if nobody ever bought it, what if nobody liked it, what if, what if...? So I have decided that the only way to do this is to do my best, not to make it perfect. I may fail, but at least I have tried. Otherwise I will never know.

I love how this lesson applies to other areas in my life as well. I have thought about starting my own business and have spent countless hours perfecting a business plan, which is good in its own right, but I think a part of the excess hours was the perfectionist in me holding me back in fear of failure. And so, I am now getting ready for and preparing to start taking more risks in my life. I am hopeful that the results will be worth it.

June 22

Recently, a wonderful opportunity has arisen for me to volunteer on the committee of the Brain Tumour Foundation of Canada's Brain-WAVE program. This is a support program for families with a child with a brain tumor. Through the program, BrainWAVE offers families the opportunity to connect with other families in a similar situation and to obtain much-needed support, information and education. They need volunteers on the committee that organizes their events in British Columbia each year.

I thought this would be a great way for me to give back, since I have not been able to do my fundraising. This will be a perfect way for me to channel my energy. One thing I know is that it is important for me to find the right things to channel my energy into. I think at this point, the combination of working with an organization such as the Brain Tumour Foundation, and directly meeting and helping families who have children with brain tumors, is a good fit for me physically and mentally. The time will come when I am able to return to fundraising as well, but for now, this is my way to give back.

I attended my first event with them up Grouse Mountain this weekend and found it inspirational and uplifting. Meeting the other volunteers and the many families, connecting with them and hearing their stories, brought home the essence of why I am so grateful I volunteered.

I have come to realize that volunteering is a two way street. It is first and foremost about giving—giving of your time, effort and compassion. But there is also the more indirect aspect of receiving—receiving the joy of being able to give your time, effort and compassion to others without any compensation, just out of the goodness of your heart. Receiving acceptance by the families as a survivor, when they asked about why I joined the BrainWAVE programme and I told them I had had a brain tumor and surgery and wanted to give back now that I had recovered.

The compassion I received from the families was humbling. This compassion from families who themselves were still struggling on a daily basis was so strong and kind; it is this type of paying it forward that makes our lives more rich and memorable.

Twenty

In the Flow

July 14

Today, I received a call from the British Columbia Ministry of Health. At first I had no idea what it was about until it dawned on me, it was in relation to the out-of-country claim I had put in for my surgical expenses in the United States. This has been a long process as it was initially denied, based off the fact I should have had the surgery done locally. I sent a letter back to them saying I had a complaint into the College of Physicians and Surgeons of British Columbia and would send them the response once I have received it, which I had done. The Ministry of Health had now reviewed my case again and were going to reimburse me for all my surgical claims. This was fantastic news! This left me feeling validated in our pursuit of pursuing the claim for these hefty expenses. It also made me feel more confident in our health care system that through the pursuit of my complaint and filing of expense claims, I had been heard. The final chapter of this whole saga was now closed.

I still see Sophia every so often to check in. The day will come when it is no longer necessary; I feel that day is coming soon. My body is so much stronger and my mind so much more able to cope with the parameters it has had to deal with over the past two years. Without a doubt, this has been the hardest two years of my life, but at the same time it's been the most gratifying on many levels.

Once again, I had a good discussion with her about being aware of challenging my body and mind while keeping it at cruising speed. I have a tendency to push to top speed as soon as I am feeling good, and then I inevitably hit a wall. I need to really get comfortable with being at cruising speed and keep an eye on my speedometer.

I know my body and brain inside and out by now; I know and truly respect them, but still need to keep an eye on my daily and weekly schedules and not push too hard. This is not being pessimistic by any means; this is being realistic with the intention of being able to live my life to the fullest within my 'new normal.'

There is a new normal for me. I do get more tired than I used to, I do sleep more than I used to, and this it is what it is. But it is not worse, it's just different. That is all.

Work is going well and the difference between April and now is very noticeable. I am still not able to work the hours I would have been able to. My GP and I have figured out that this may only be possible once the summer is over. But my stamina is greatly improved.

I have found that the big key to daily success is being aware of my triggers, just like a typical migraine patient would. Except for me I don't get a migraine, I get a vestibular effect. The result is dis-equilibrium and I feel like I am losing my balance.

My triggers are not enough sleep, too much stress, nuts, caffeine, chocolate and alcohol. Oh, and I take my medication and natural migraine supplement every day, and keep exercising. I think that is not a bad situation to be in. If that is my lot in life to carry after brain surgery, I am okay with that.

The other important thing to be aware of is my threshold. Your threshold is all about knowing your body and where it stands in this moment. Did you have enough sleep the night before? Are you stressed at the moment? What is your threshold today? If you have slept well and are not stressed and avoiding all trigger foods, your threshold is probably low, so you could indulge in a cup of decent caffeinated coffee. But if you have not slept well and have a stressful situation at work, grabbing that cup of coffee just because you feel you need it might send you over the edge. This explains why one day a cup of coffee has no effect and another day it gives you a tremendous migraine (or, in my situation, makes me feel like I am on a ship in a storm).

So, finding the balance for me and being aware of my body's needs and status each day is important to how I fare by the end of the week —this is no change, as this is how it has been since the surgery. Respecting my body is the key.

August 25

Slowly but surely, the heat of the summer is fading out of the days. We have had one of the best summers I can remember since we have lived here: almost four months of warm days and blue skies; only two or three days of rain. It has been amazing.

We have truly embraced all the days of sun by being outside biking, at the beach, on a road trip to Oregon, a weekend to Whistler. We even bought Aiden a kayak this summer. He has loved the feeling of independence on the water with his friends, who also got their first kayaks. The Three Musketeers have headed off on their intrepid adventures

.t our local beach many a time over the past summer weeks. He has had so much fun that Marchand and I have bought our own kayaks to join in on the action. I remembered so clearly that wonderful sense of childlike adventure when Aiden and I went kayaking together at the end of last summer, I cannot wait to recreate that feeling.

I have also started to meditate again. With the re-invigoration of my body, my Type A personality is rising to the surface and trying to put its foot on the gas. I now know that I can really only operate on cruising speed most of the time, with a few hours of acceleration in between. No more acceleration all the time, as I used to be able to do. I remembered how well my brain responded to meditation after my surgery so I have decided to try it out again. This time I am working with the same empowerment group, SPARK creations, on their FLOW program. Learning to be at peace, embrace my soul and be at my optimum. It's perfect timing for me as I embrace my new energy again and try to balance it all out.

I have set a clear intention as I enter this new chapter. "To be still, and give myself permission to be so." I have always struggled with the concept of being still, probably because I have always been so busy. Maybe I am always so busy because I am a perfectionist and not willing to fail and let go. After my surgery, I had to be still because my body could not actually be any other way. Now that I am so much better, I need to remember how to be still and actually have to learn how to practice it for the sake of my brain and body, as I still need that sense of peace and calm each day. I think most of us do and should do.

The meditation I am doing each night before I go to bed has been remarkable. I have been using the same phone app again by Jon Kabat-Zinn, one of the pioneers in the therapeutic applications of mindfulness, and my sleep has been that much deeper. That may be one of the reasons I have been experiencing an energy growth over the past weeks as well. I have been doing a bit of research into mind-

176

fulness and today I listened to a very interesting documentary about it on the radio. A vast amount of scientific literature supports its positive impact on the brain, mind, body, level of focus, stress, even areas such as compassion and the ability for individuals with chronic conditions to reintegrate into everyday life.

Along with its positive impact on my sleep and energy levels, I have noticed a gentler and kinder impact on my person as well. There really is a mind-body connection.

August 31

Another year. I almost cannot believe that another year has passed me by. The thirty-first of August is here again. To most people this would seem bizarre, to take note of the fact that this was two years to the day that I was having brain surgery and in ICU. But to the patient in that ICU bed that day, although it fades farther away into the past, it is still in their memory. There is something about having had brain surgery that stays with you.

The first year is a big milestone, as often that first year of recovery is longer and more arduous than expected. The second year was not what I expected. I thought I was good to go after the first year, but then did a little hop skip and a jump backwards. I am glad to report that as I approach my second brainiversary I feel strong, both mentally and physically. I now know my new normal and see it in a positive light. This is me. I love the new me.

Yes, I went through a grieving process for the old me who could work endless hours and do anything I wanted to. But I love the new me for the lessons I have learned that have shaped and added to the person that I am today. I love the new me for the appreciation of small things I never before have felt to this extent. I love the new me for the respect and gratitude I have for my body and brain, after all it has been through. I love the new me for the way in which I love my husband, son and family in more ways than before. Yes, I am different and changed from the old me; this is perhaps not noticeable to anyone from the outside—perhaps only to those closest to me. But I am stronger in so many ways than I was before.

Everyone's journey and story through a major surgery or health condition is different. Mine is like my own pair of shoes. The size may fit someone else but may feel a bit tight or uncomfy on the toes or ankle. But I have decided to share it regardless because there are some aspects of it that will ring true to someone else and that part of the shoe will fit.

How my fundraising will continue in the future I am not one hundred percent sure, what I do know is that I have found a heart warming and gratifying way to give back through the BrainWAVE programme and that is key. Direct contact with children and families who have been through a similar journey and being a part of organizing events that bring a sense of fun and support to their lives is a great opportunity.

In recognition of this two-year milestone, I have decided to create a mosaic. My mosaic is made up of small glass pieces glued to a rock in the shape of two feet, which are truly symbolic of my journey, one step after another, always moving forward. It's also apt for where it is going to be placed. Since the seawall has been an integral part of my recovery, both mind and body, I decided to set my mosaic in the rocks at the seawall walk.

Many mosaics already exist on the seawall rocks and I think mine will be happy there with the ocean breeze, seals and seagulls. So, the two feet that I created are a gentle tribute to those who walk the seawall every day, with their own thoughts or with their friends and families, to enjoy the beautiful scenery and splendor.

For me, it is recognition of the first day I walked that seawall two months after my surgery, just for five minutes each way, and the euphoric feeling of achievement I felt that day. I will never forget it. It is a reminder of how far we can come, and also how important the small things in life really are.

And so with this soul searching and recent journey of discovery, I have also realized that the chapters of my life are going to be written on a continuous basis. This book will never have a true ending. I could probably write another book on the next stage of my life, but for now, the saying "Life is a journey and not a destination" could not be truer. I have discovered that my life is not about finding myself, it really is all about creating myself, as I read in a quote today.

My life is in my hands. There are great possibilities ahead. Even as I read this last chapter now, it brings tears to my eyes as I know: I am blessed today. I am truly grateful. Two steps forward I go, as I embrace the next chapter of my life.

Twenty One

Being a Parent

I WANTED TO WRITE THESE WORDS FOR THOSE OF YOU WHO may have young children when you are first diagnosed with a health condition. It adds another layer to the paradigm. My first thoughts after diagnosis were of my son and husband. Would I live to see my son grow up? When I got home after being in the ER, Aiden was sound asleep. I remember watching him sleeping, only four years old and all pink-cheeked, oblivious to the goings-on around him. My heart literally felt sore, almost shattered, inside my chest. As parents, we will do anything to protect our children; it really is a primal instinct.

Here are some of my lessons:

Telling your children

Whether and how to broach your health condition with your children is a very personal decision. It depends on the age of the children, and how much they can take on board.

Children differ greatly in their individual natures as well as in their maturity. They seem to be very matter-of-fact about a lot of things of this nature. It's similar to the 'sex' talk—they take on as much as their brains and emotional state and maturity are able to at the time. The rest tends to glide over their heads and seems irrelevant. It's almost a protective mechanism.

Aiden was only four years old when everything first happened. He was too young to really understand events, so we did not discuss my tumor with him. He just knew that Mom was sick and would be at home, getting better.

From a practical perspective, Aiden knew from preschool what an emergency looked like and how to dial 911. After my diagnosis we reinforced this with him, just to be on the safe side. In August 2012, when I started to get acutely ill and developed hydrocephalus, we were transparent with Aiden about any tests I was having. But we did not show fear to him; rather we told him that we were doing tests to ensure that everything was okay.

When I was finally diagnosed with hydrocephalus and we had to leave for the surgery in Baltimore, Aiden was six years old. He was more able to grasp what was going on around him, but was still only a young child. We did tell him that Mom was going to have surgery to make her better, but didn't provide specific detail.

Hospital visits

Looking back, it amazes me at how resilient kids are. To this day, if we ask Aiden what one of his best holidays was, he will reply, "Baltimore, when Mom had brain surgery." Who would have thought? I still giggle about it. He had Granny there, he stayed in a great hotel, which had a pool, and he went to cool museums, had cool food and missed school. Awesome! Aiden and I did not see each other for four days as he could not visit the ICU. On the day I did walk out the ICU to see him, he was terrified and jumped into Marchand's arms. I realized that the reality was too much for him.

So perhaps taking kids to the hospital to visit, especially really young kids, should be discussed. Not many adults, let alone kids, feel comfortable in an ICU setting. It can be traumatic to see a parent attached to IVs or things they do not understand. Keeping in touch by phone is a good option. Hearing mom or dad's voice reassures children that everything is all right. Aiden did not come back to the hospital again, even when I was readmitted with meningitis—it was just easier to speak on the phone, and better for him in the long run.

Your children's emotions

One thing we did notice during my surgery and re-admittance to hospital, then coming home and going back to school, was that Aiden got more nervous than usual when he sensed change was coming. This made total sense, given everything he had been through in the past month. So, we took extra care to be mindful of this over the next while and with time, he was back to his normal self.

Children sometimes react very differently to how we would expect them to react in these types of situations because we are expecting an adult reaction. So keep an eye out for changes in behavior—this could be your child's way of expressing their emotions, and it might not be what you expect.

Post-surgical changes

For me, as a parent, the bigger challenge was actually in the recovery after surgery and not the diagnosis. The immense and sometime crippling fatigue and prolonged recovery was hard, as I struggled to get back to being a mom and a wife. For the first two months post-surgery, when I was heavily fatigued, I needed help fetching him from school and caring for him. It also meant explaining to a six-year-old what it meant for Mom to not be firing on all cylinders. Impatience and frustration were common feelings, and I had to ask for Aiden's help to get through it all.

It was important for him to know that it was not his fault that Mom turned into a 'monster' by 5pm—her body was just so tired, and small things were really sapping her energy. Organizing play dates with good friends after school or on the weekend was an integral part to helping Aiden feel like life was good and things were moving forward. It also made me feel better, as I knew he was happy. At the innocent age of six, life is simple. The more things moved forward in a routine, the better things went for everyone.

I cannot deny there were moments when I lost it as a parent. When Aiden threw comments back to me, that cut deep. There were times when the exhaustion and frustration of my recovery went down to my bones and barely allowed me to function, let alone be the loving and patient mom I needed to be. I knew Aiden resented my brain surgery and my fatigue, especially when I could not keep up with his demands and do things that other parents could do.

My words of advice for parents who are recovering from brain surgery, or major surgery of any kind, is to find small moments and relish them. There may be many times you feel inadequate as a mom or a dad or caregiver, times when your fatigue overwhelms you. You might become grumpier through frustration or impatience. By the end of the day, you might even feel guilty.

Take five minutes each day when you do have the energy to revel in the love you have with your child. Just be with them and do whatever it is that they want to do. Let them feel all that attention just for them, in that moment, so that when it starts to unravel at the end of the day, they remember subconsciously the moment you shared.

Also, find a few things that you can do with them, e.g. build a puzzle, read a book—things that do not fracture your energy. Another lesson for me was to ensure that I made peace with Aiden at the end of each day. Fatigue meant that my tolerance level after surgery was very different. Sometimes, by the end of the day I felt like I had left the day on a bad note with Aiden—in my mind, not necessarily in reality.

Wipe the slate clean

Because I went to bed so early, almost straight after he did, I missed out on that incredibly special moment I used to relish, that moment of peeking in on him sleeping. Even now that is one of the most special parts of my day. It is the moment I remember what a miracle he is and how very blessed we are, and it fills my heart up for the next day. No matter what the day held for us both, this is the clean slate, the white flag. The next day dawns anew. So, I make sure now to always go in and wipe the slate clean, and be thankful for my miracle and kiss his soft cheek goodnight.

Confidence in your parenting

My confidence as a mom has definitely been rocked during this adventure. I had to rely on other people to be 'mom' to Aiden for at least the first two months post op. When I was back in that role yet struggling with extreme fatigue and the resulting irritability and impatience, at times I felt like I was an incompetent mom. Not that I could not look after him; that was not the issue. It was more that I couldn't always be the mom I wanted to be: patient, kind and understanding. That was hard for me, especially by the end of the day.

I found initially that I would get unusually stressed about play dates. I have realized that a lot of this is related to the fact that in the initial months, I had to rely on so many other people to take on tasks I used to consider easy to do and just part of every day. My stamina and faith in my abilities had been taxed so many times that I questioned my ability with certain things. I also found that I was oversensitive to Aiden's antics as an energetic seven-year-old. Because my energy levels were so linked to my patience and tolerance as a mom, I overreacted to him being naughty, trying to protect myself from getting fatigued. I am now aware of this being a negative issue, and one that I used as a coping strategy. If Aiden was playing up, I would rather pack up and leave than battle it out—it was too tiring for me. I found it better to be open with other moms around me when I felt I was getting oversensitive about his antics. I let them know that I hope I didn't seem irritable or oversensitive, but that my brain sometimes struggled to find the balance between managing my energy levels and being a mom. I did this not to gain sympathy, but to inform them and decrease my own stress as well.

As a side note, I found that around one year post surgery, the issues with stress and confidence improved dramatically. By eighteen months post-op, things were mostly back to normal. I think this has a lot to do with the decreased fatigue and improved short-term memory that came with passing that 'one year' post-op mark. My local neurosurgeon said it would make a huge difference, and he was right!

With my second round of medical appointments and my potential second brain surgery, we were very open with Aiden about what was going on. I think this worked well, as he was now seven-and-a-half years old.

One day I was on the phone to the doctor in the United States and they told me I might not be able to get an appointment for three months. I told them I was not able to work due to my symptoms and, after completing my call, I put down the phone and wept in sheer frustration. Aiden came up to me and put his arms around me and gave me a hug, saying, "It's okay, Mom, it will be alright." I was taken aback by his empathy and felt humbled by his maturity. Your children can surprise you in the oddest moments.

Connections

Looking back, I think the best thing is to be as honest as you feel necessary, keeping in mind your child's capability to accept the facts. Love them, respect them and talk to them while still keeping the adult role model present for them to see that someone is in control. This is important and offers them a sense of stability and safety in the home environment. When you are not having a good day, they may surprise you with how much they understand and empathize. At the same time, they are simple beings. Depending on their age, they may not need a plethora of information, so tell them things only as they need to know. For me, the physical connection was challenging as my body was weak and fatigued. Remember to give those hugs and kisses and maintain the physical connection as much as possible if that is an important part of your relationship. I found months later that it was as if with the surgery, this connection had been severed as well. With time and my energy, this returned and with it my son's realization that mom was still here.

At the end of the day, let us be grateful for these wonderful beings.

Twenty Two

BEING A PATIENT

On a positive level, I have learnt to:

- Be my body's own advocate

- Love and appreciate the small things in life and be grateful for them

- Live each day as it comes

- Learn to put things into perspective

- Know and truly respect my body

Notes to self

These are some notes I made for myself during my recovery—my learning points—which I have printed out and put in my office as a reminder to myself. I thought they may be useful to share.

1. Be your own advocate! If something does not feel right, seek medical attention until they can resolve the issue and you feel comfortable and adequately satisfied with the resolution.

2. Take each day as it comes. It could even mean take each hour as it comes, especially in the beginning. Know that each person has a unique experience with the condition and also post-surgery.

   a. Look at your days and week ahead and make sure it is not chaos, with no time for quiet for you and your brain.

3. Listen to your body and your brain. Mental fatigue can be as crippling as physical fatigue. They are closely linked and feed off each other.

4. There may be a 'new normal' you need to find. It does not mean a 'lesser normal' but something new—and it could be better! Mine is.

5. Identify the triggers that may cause you to feel fatigued or off-kilter. Try to minimize your exposure to them. If you have no option, be mindful that it may fatigue you, and plan how to work with it.

6. As a parent, spouse, partner, or in any other relationship, try to find five minutes each day when you are feeling at your best, when you can connect with this person and create positive memories. Store them up.

7. Keep an objective 'eye on yourself.' As you get stronger, keep track of any negative behaviors that are able to morph back into positive behaviors e.g. mommy monster. It is easy to get stuck in a rut. Remind yourself, as you get stronger, to 'check in' on yourself regularly.

8. Make peace with yourself and with others about your abilities. This may still need to happen long after you first think it would.

9. Once you are stronger, think about whether you are pre-conditioning your mind about what your body can do, given the

past experience you have had. Can you try things again and see if you are able to do them now? You might surprise your-self!

10. Know that you might look and seem to be totally recovered on the outside, but on the inside you might still be recovering, and that some parts of you might never recover to the exact same person you were before surgery. This is okay. Don't run from it: embrace it.

What I asked my neurosurgeon about my condition after I was diagnosed

I found it useful to keep a list of questions and a diary of my symptoms in the beginning, after my diagnosis, so that when I saw my doctor, I had all the details in one place. Also, it is useful to take someone with you to see your neurosurgeon/neurologist. You might forget exactly what the doctor said, or forget to ask one very important question.

This is a list of questions I put together in the beginning, when I saw the various specialists:

☐ How much experience do you have with this condition? i.e. how many patients do you see with colloid cysts each year?

☐ How many patients with my condition have you operated on?

☐ What is your current opinion on treatment of the condition?

☐ Does this opinion go along with what happens worldwide?

☐ Do I need MRIs to monitor the condition? If so, how often? How does this match worldwide opinion?

☐ How do you determine when to do surgery?

☐ At what size do most people need the colloid cyst removed?

Surgical questions

☐ How long would I wait until surgery, if you recommend it?

☐ How long does the operation take?

☐ What type of operation do you perform?

☐ Time in hospital and which wards (ICU)

☐ Post-surgical rehabilitation, if required

☐ Medications

☐ Risks during surgery

☐ Key challenges after surgery

- Acute (in hospital and after discharge)
- Long-term

☐ How long does it take to go back to work/school?

☐ How long to get 'back to normal'?

☐ Post op follow up

- MRIs
- Neurosurgical appointments
- Rehab appointments

What to do before surgery?

This is the type of information I would have liked to have before surgery—it is not a medical opinion. Unfortunately, because my surgery was more unplanned, I did not have much time to prepare, so we did not get around to doing all of these things.

1. Ensure the 'house is in order'. Meaning if you have bills to pay or things to sort out, put it in place before the surgery.

2. Think of all the things you normally do each day and allocate them to someone else, if they still need to happen: e.g. work responsibilities, walking the dog, paying the bills, taking care of children. Let them lapse if you can.

3. Make a few meals and freeze them or reach out to friends and family to bring over meals for the first few weeks. By the end of each day you might not be up to cooking a gourmet meal, but you will need good nutrition to recover.

4. Write a list of all your important accounts and their passwords. Your brain will be focusing on healing, not remembering the multitude of passwords we all have to keep these days!

5. Ensure you have a power of attorney in place if necessary, and create or update your will. This may seem morbid, but any surgery, even minor surgery, carries risk.

6. If you have kids, organize some fun play dates for them after your surgery so you know they are happy and having fun. It allows you to relax when you know the kids are taken care of.

7. Chat to your close friends and loved ones about your recovery. Let them know that it may take some time before you are back to doing everything. Let them know you have no idea what it will be like for you and that each day will be one step at a time.

8. Figure out how and to whom information will be sent out about your surgery and post-op recovery. People will always want to know that you are safely out of the operating theatre and making a good recovery, but you don't want to be inundated with calls in the acute stages.

9. If you have any form of disability insurance/critical illness or income protection insurance and intend to exercise it after surgery, this is the time to look into what needs to be done with regards paperwork and applying for it.

What to take to hospital?

1. Super comfy pajamas and socks

   - You will most likely be in hospital gear for a day or so after the surgery, then you can change into something more comfy and familiar. There is nothing like your own PJ's.

   - Sturdy pair of slippers for your 'walks' through the ICU when you are getting up and mobile.

2. Toiletries

   - Take some nice lip balm or Vaseline, as your lips get so dry, especially after surgery.

   - Hand cream.

   - Take your prescription medications to the hospital and they will tell you what you can or cannot take.

3. Neck pillow

   - I found this invaluable. My mom said to take my travel neck pillow into hospital and it was great—just another position you can get your head into post op.

4. Reading material

   - A book may be hard going after surgery, depending on how tired you are. So a magazine may be nice to glance at if your body and brain allow.

5. Notepad and pen

   - It's nice to write something down if you want to ask the doctor or nurse a question, or anything else that comes to mind. Don't tax your brain with trying to remember it, or being frustrated when you can't.

6. Something personal

- It is nice to take in something personal and comforting to hospital, but not anything that can get lost or that is valuable.

- For a child, a nice stuffy toy is lovely. However, note, that I was very happy with the stuffy bunny my Mom bought me for my stay in hospital too!

What to expect after surgery

This is information I think may be useful to have after surgery, it is definitely not a medical opinion. Please seek medical advice if you are concerned about <u>any</u> of your symptoms and follow any advice given to you by your medical team.

This is the hardest part to write, as everyone has such different experiences after brain surgery (or after any surgery). My list includes questions asked on a regular basis in our group as well. I have found, however, that often after any surgery, the advice you are given regarding recovery may differ in its thoroughness, regardless of where you had the surgery. So, here is my two cents worth, based on my individual experience:

1. **My stages of recovery**

    a. *Acute recovery (<3 months)*

        - Rest, rest and more rest!

            - The extreme fatigue I felt in the acute phase took me (and us all) completely by surprise. I did not realize that I would be sleeping for anywhere up to sixteen hours a day for the first four weeks. I would nap two or three times a day and sometimes just lie in bed and read (if I could manage that part). Things like going for a doctor's visit, or chatting to someone for too long definitely needed a nap afterwards.

- *Rule of thumb*: Sleep till your body cannot sleep any more! It all benefits the brain and your healing process. There seems to be no time limit on this phase of sleeping.

- Doctors visits

  - Write down any questions for your doctor in a notebook so when you get there, you can remember them all (my memory was not stellar in the acute phase)!

  - Have someone go with you for your first few visits. I found this useful so that I could remember exactly what was said to me, or if I forgot to ask an important question I had been meaning to ask.

- Medications

  - Post surgery there seemed to be a never-ending medication regime, from Keppra to dexamethasone to anti-nausea pills. Some post-op medications can increase fatigue, but they are necessary, so it is a wicked cycle. Take everything that is prescribed according to your doctor's recommendations and call them if you have any questions.

  - Some of the medications made me sleep, some made me stay awake, some gave me mood swings and some made me eat like a beast. But they all served their purpose and pulled me through my recovery, so I took them all as prescribed. That is the main thing!

- *Rule of thumb*: Keep track of what you need to take and when (or even better, get a caregiver to do so). Keep a diary so you know if you have taken your meds or not. Believe me, you might not be able to remember, and under or overdosing is not an option!

b. *Recovery (3-12 months)*

- In general, I found this went in ups and downs or two steps forward and one step back.

- Be patient. Be patient with your body and your brain. On the days that you are feeling good, don't try to run a marathon. Embrace the feeling, but don't overdo it. You will get there through baby steps, and you and your body will be happier for it.

- I still had to nap every lunch time until I was twelve months post op. Even at eighteen months post-op, I sometimes needed a nap if it had been a busy weekend or day. I have learned to be in tune with my body and know its limits. Napping means my brain was in need of a 'recharge' in order for it to perform at its optimum.

- Continue to respect your body (and brain!) for what it has been through and know it will come right. It might be slightly different from before but if you embrace that, rather than fight it, the path is that much easier.

2. **Hair or no hair?**

   a. To be honest, this did not cross my mind, given the unplanned nature of my operation.

   b. Depending on the type of surgery you have, you may have a neat small incision-patch behind your hairline or you could have a more shaved appearance if you had a full craniotomy. If you have enough time, ask your surgeon what to expect.

   c. If you usually get your hair colored, and if you have time to do so before surgery, do it. It might be a while before you can do so again, and post-op you might not want to expose your scar to chemicals for a while.

   d. Keep a beanie/toque handy, especially if you have surgery in fall or winter. There is something very comforting about having your head wrapped warm and tight. I slept with a beanie for months after my surgery and even now, when the weather changes and my head aches, it is very comforting to put my beanie on.

   e. Your hair will look bizarre after surgery, as it may have been wrapped up tight in a bandage for days. I looked like I had had a perm and was a brunette (and I am a blonde) from all the surgical disinfectant they had put on my scalp. The picture my husband took of me was a classic. The first hair wash is memorable to this day!

3. **Sleep**

   a. The amount of sleep my body needed to recover was astounding. No-one really explained to me that I

would sleep ten hours or more at night and then fluc-
tuate between napping and being awake for an hour
at a time in the beginning.

b. Given that the way your brain heals is to sleep and
switch off all non-essential functions, lots of sleeping
in the beginning makes sense. You may even find your
body still needs to nap up to one year or more after
surgery. Everyone is different in what they need.

c. I only stopped napping at lunchtime about one year
post op.

d. You may also suffer from insomnia depending on
your post-surgery medications. I found that the dexamethasone gave me insomnia at night and so did my
elevated cortisol, even though my brain just wanted
to sleep.

4. **Pain**

a. Post op

- I was told prior to my surgery that the brain
itself has no pain receptors, so the pain
would be more from the incision and craniotomy.

- Indeed, the actual pain from the surgery
was real but not overbearing. I had oxycodone for the headache (ache in the head,
literally) immediately post-op. When I was
discharged, I had Tylenol for the pain and
oxycodone if things got really unbearable. I
rarely had to use the latter.

- I had pain post-op from the IV lines and
arterial line in my arms.

b. Headaches

- Because I never had headaches or migraines until I was diagnosed with a colloid cyst, I thought they would just go away after surgery.

- Unfortunately, I still get migraines, even two years post op. It is just part of life. I have my daily preventative migraine medication and know that extreme fatigue and some foods will set it off. I just work with it instead of against it.

c. Pain around scar and incision site

- The strangest thing was when, about two weeks after surgery, I actually 'felt' my head. It felt like it had craters in it, bumps, craters and ridges. Wow! This was an interesting adventure. Even two years out, it sometimes feels like it may have changed shape a bit, or an area might irritate me for a day or two.

- As I continued into my recovery and the area around my incision started to 'wake-up,' I had feelings from pain to numbness to just plain old aching. This seems to be what most people encounter, but obviously contact your doctor if anything seems out of the norm.

- Even now, cold and changes in weather make my head ache. I feel I can predict a weather change myself! So a beanie is still very useful if it is cold.

d. Neck and Back Pain

- I think given the weird positions you are often put in for the actual brain surgery, sometimes your neck or back may feel a bit painful and stiff during the acute recovery period.

- Also, if you are less mobile during your recovery, your body tends to feel it. If permitted, a gentle short walk each day is a good option. Walk with someone down the road and back, just to keep your body moving. It will also be good for the soul and, as you see yourself get stronger, good for the motivation.

- A hot or cold pack on my neck or back was useful as well.

- I started to see my massage therapist and chiropractor after consulting with my neurosurgeon and this helped alleviate the pain.

5. **Driving**

di. Depending on where you live, some countries/states have laws which do not allow people to drive for up to a year after brain surgery. Check with your doctor if there is any such legal issue in your jurisdiction.

dii. I was given clearance to drive once I was off all pain medications and anti-seizure medications, and when I felt able to do so. This was about two months post op.

diii. I actually didn't drive until four weeks after I was cleared to do so. I did so when it felt right to do it, and I started off slowly.

d. It is not only your life and but also others who are involved when you drive. Make sure you are ready and feel competent. I held off on driving long distances or driving at night for a while longer.

6. Memory

a. Well yes, that topic of short–term memory is tricky, as it seems a lot of people with colloid cysts suffer from memory issues before surgery. I did, but not in any extreme way, apart from when I developed hydrocephalus.

b. After surgery, I felt like my short-term memory was not great. I compensated by ensuring I kept note of things I needed to do, lists and so forth to keep the wheels moving. I felt like a goldfish in many moments! This passes, with time.

c. I also started playing brain games such as Lumosity on my iPhone to challenge my brain and give it some homework. I still challenge myself now to remember what I have to do the next day, instead of just looking at my calendar. One-year post op I noticed a big improvement in my short-term memory.

d. My long-term memory still has gaps in it even to this day.

7. Moods

a. Fatigue, and frustration with the fatigue and prolonged recovery, can make one feel more impatient and 'fragile' at the end of the day. Mood swings can also be related to the extreme change that has happened, as well as to medications. Your body and mind are adjusting to just having had brain surgery!

b. Keeping an eye on your moods and state of mind is a good thing. Keep an open channel of communication with your family physician about this if you feel you are struggling more than you anticipated. Seeing a therapist or psychologist is another tool to assist in recovery after such a surgery.

8. Stamina

a. As you progress in your recovery, you will hopefully notice changes in your stamina and ability to do things. It may be something small like being able to climb the stairs at home without feeling exhausted.

b. If you feel your stamina is not where you think it should be, chat to your family physician. Major surgery can have an impact on the way your body functions.

9. Stress/Lack of confidence

a. My ability to deal with stress and my general lack of confidence has been a challenge since my surgery. This was not an issue for me before my surgery.

b. A good friend said to me, we all head to the doctor for a sore throat but yet when we are under extreme stress we never seek help to chat to someone about it.

c. If it means seeing a therapist/psychologist, or whatever it takes for you to feel more confident in your abilities as well as less stressed, look into it. I started seeing a clinical therapist and it made a tremendous difference to me. It taught me to be more in tune with my body as well as my mind, a great life lesson in so many ways.

10. Vertigo and imbalance

    a. Having struggled with vertigo prior to surgery, I thought it would be a thing of the past after surgery, but it was not.

    b. Speak to your family physician about options to assist you if you find that vertigo is impacting your daily life. It can be debilitating and incredibly tiring.

    c. Vestibular physiotherapy helped me tremendously; over months my brain learned to counteract the 'false messages' it was getting regarding my imbalance. This website offers a good explanation of vestibular rehabilitation therapy: https://vestibular.org/understanding-vestibular-disorder/treatment/treatment-detail-page

11. Return to work/school

If you know the date of your surgery and are able to prepare for it in advance, speak to your work place in advance about your return-to-work plan. Discuss with them the fact that you are not 100 percent certain about the time frame of your recovery. Most neurosurgeons will be able to give you an estimated date for return to work, and that will be important for your workplace to know.

The most important part of your discussion will be regarding gradual entry back to the workplace. You may be able to go straight back to normal work hours; however, it might be a better option to start with a gradual entry. This may mean part-time hours for a week and gradually increasing your hours until you are back at your original schedule.

Thes ame discussion or rationale should take place for a return to school or university. A work setting usually involves a high level of focus and attention, which places high demands on the brain.

This can result in a very tired person, either half way through the day or at the end of the day. Keep the channels of communication open between you and your work colleagues or boss on your progress on reintegrating at work—it is important to your success!

Twenty Three

BEING YOUR BODY'S OWN ADVOCATE

I WRITE THIS CHAPTER TO CELEBRATE MY TEN-YEAR BRAINI-versary. This a milestone in not only my life but also for those around me.

To this day, I can vividly remember being diagnosed in the emergency room, in my backless blue gown, as the cold rush of air passed over my skin. Those words, "you have a brain tumor" are forever etched in my mind and have created a line in the sand of the 'before' and 'after' in our lives.

I did not realize when I was diagnosed that I was being catapulted into one of the most complex systems in the world, the health care system. I was no longer a routine patient but one with multiple appointments, multiple medications, and multiple specialists.

Navigating the health care system at this level required a degree of ownership, of administration and management. Health care Navigation 101 was not a course that I had taken.

My patient journey over the past decade has been touched and positively impacted by many amazing and committed individuals working within this complex system. At the same time, my life has also hung in the balance and been negatively impacted due to the complexity of the system.

The reason I sit and write these words is because of my hope that each and every person who reads them will realize that their health is too important to take lightly. There are ways that each of us can take responsibility, be proactive and put our health in our own hands. We might save a life – our own, or the life of someone we love.

This, however, is easier said than done. It is no easy task.

It's hard to be a manager, administrator and a patient or caregiver all at the same time, especially when you are at your most vulnerable.

I always thought that the health care system would sort everything out for me, be in control and have my back. I soon realized; this was not the case. I was wrong.

There were too many silos of good people working in opposite directions. I was the only one living my reality, 24/7, and knew the intricacies of my patient journey. Health care systems are complex and overburdened for both patients and the people working within them. Mistakes can happen. We are only human after all.

During my patient journey, I quickly realized the importance of finding an approach to help me manage my health and health care. Our life was turned upside down following my brain tumor diagnosis, and the feelings of uncertainty, powerlessness and fear were very real. There is something to be said for having a lifeline to keep you grounded. Mine was ensuring that I was in control of my health. This probably came from my training as a product manager. When uncertainty arises, make a plan! Well, this plan ended up saving my life.

My plan was a T.E.A.M. Approach. Learn to **T**rack, **E**ducate, **A**sk and **M**anage. Gather your support groups, families, and health care teams at your side. Today, I share this approach with you.

TRACK

From the start, it is important to track and keep records of everything relevant to your patient journey. This could be related to your medical history, symptom tracking, medication information, health records, and copies of test results. I have a big red binder that I started after my diagnosis, to chronicle the story of my brain and I. Today, as a patient with other chronic conditions, I have other binders holding the stories of my other journeys.

EDUCATE

Being an informed and educated—but not overwhelmed—individual is essential to making informed decisions. Education allows patients and caregivers to participate in discussions with their health care teams. Becoming educated and accessing and understanding information in an easily digested, reliable format is key. Ask your health care team for the best place to find information on your health condition, so that you know it is reliable and accurate.

ASK

Asking questions can be challenging, as it requires courage. However, asking questions is fundamental to the success of the T.E.A.M Approach. You can start by asking questions such as: *Why, what if, and how can we do this together?* This can help open communication between you and your health care professional and team.

MANAGE

Teams become effective with good management, and the same is true for health care. Managing helps set objectives for an individual's health care by asking questions such as: What do I want for my health care, from my medical team, and from the doctor's appointment I am about to attend? Setting objectives can help remove some of the emotional aspects from the individual's condition and help them regain control of uncertain situations. *For me personally, adding in the management part to my health diagnosis helped me gain more control and feel less powerless.*

SUPPORT GROUPS

To 'support' means to keep from falling. This is an apt descriptor for a good support group, consisting of individuals who are brought together because of a common interest (or health condition) and share experiences, lessons, and connections. Support groups for health-related conditions can literally keep you from falling at times.

I know. I joined an online Facebook brain tumor support group straight after my diagnosis and an in-person group later. The people in this group have been with me through diagnosis, surgery, recovery and more. It's not that my family has not been amazingly supportive and loving—not at all! It's just that to talk to people who are walking in the same shoes is sometimes easier.

HEALTH CARE TEAMS

With any health care diagnosis, it is often the doctor who delivers the words that can change our lives, our outlook on our health, and the way we think about things. It is critical that we connect, communicate, and collaborate with our health care team. We need to gather our health care teams by our side, ask questions and ask them to support us as we are becoming more active in our health care.

FAMILIES & FRIENDS

Being an immigrant, I am the first to know that not everyone has immediate family around that they are able to count on—for whatever reason that may be. It's the connection and the support that comes from familiarity that's important. If that comes from friends or colleagues, then our friends become our family. Having emotional, and sometimes physical, support is integral to the patient journey. Our care partners can come in all shapes and forms. They say, "it takes a village" and this could not be more true—because together we are stronger. Look for opportunities to reach out to family and friends—the power of community can be humbling.

Just by reading this chapter, you are already taking steps to be proactive and look for ways to put your health in your own hands. You know that your health is too important to take lightly.

Health care systems all over the world are complex and overburdened for both patients and health care teams. Mistakes can happen. We are only human, after all.

Remember: because this IS the reality of life, you need a T.E.A.M Approach. Learn to Track, Educate, Ask and Manage. Gather your support groups, family, and health care teams at your side.

You might save a life—your own, or the life of someone you love.

Find more resources
and information at

WWW.TWOSTEPS.CA

EPILOGUE

September

The 'circle of life' continues around me. Spring and summer have come and gone again and fall is here. I can map my last three years by the seasons. Three summers ago, I had hydrocephalus and brain surgery. Two summers ago, I finally got my strength and 'mojo' back, only to take a step backwards in the early fall. Now here I am with the heat of the summer fading out of the days and the leaves starting to fall. My body is recovered, my spirit is renewed, my medication regime is still working and I have once again learned to listen to my body, be mindful and respectful of its abilities, celebrate its achievements and be grateful for each day. For this I am happy.

I think the key lesson for me in this chapter of my life has been that no matter how many times I feel like I have fallen down, whether physi-cally or mentally, I can get up again and I will be able to get through it and go forward. I can do it. Life is an adventure every day. Some days are more challenging than others, but I am here and embracing it and loving it—Two Steps Forward I go!

Dear Reader,

I do hope you enjoyed reading Two Steps Forward – Embracing life with a brain tumor.

As a first time author, I would love any feedback you have about the book. What was the most useful thing you took away or learnt from the book - did you share anything from the book with a friend? Feel free to connect with me at claire@twosteps.ca.

I have also developed a website supporting the book where you can subscribe to my newsletter, read my blog, access resources, and much more. Hope you can visit soon: www.twosteps.ca.

I have a favor to ask of you. I would love it if you could take the time to do a book review for me, even if just two sentences. As a first time author, reviews are not easy to come by and would be greatly appreciated. All reviews help increase visibility of the book online and hopefully allow more brain tumor survivors and general readers looking for such a resource to easily find it. Here is where you can find and review my book on Amazon: www.amazon.com/author/clairesnyman

Thanks again for reading Two Steps Forward.

With gratitude,

Claire Snyman

About the Author

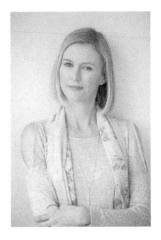

Claire Snyman, brain tumor and brain surgery survivor, releases her first book, *Two Steps Forward – Embracing life with a brain tumor* about the often-harrowing journey through life with a non-malignant brain tumor, her misdiagnosis and consequent brain surgery and recovery.

Claire is a patient experience consultant, lover of life and nature, wife and mother and loves to explore new ways of achieving balance in life. She is now an author, speaker and health care advocate, using her lived experience to increase communication and collaboration between patients, families, caregivers and the health care system.

Learn more at www.twosteps.ca

Made in United States
Orlando, FL
30 January 2023

29237391R00134